Whose Body
Is It Anyway?

Other Books by Joan Kenley

A Woman's Right to Know
Voice Power

Whose Body Is It Anyway?

Smart Alternative and Traditional Health Choices for Your Total Well-Being

Joan Kenley

with John C. Arpels, M.D.

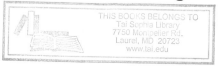
Newmarket Press
New York

Copyright © 1999 Joan Kenley

This book is published in the United States of America.
All rights reserved. This book may not be reproduced, in whole or in
part, in any form, without written permission. Inquiries should be
addressed to Permissions Department, Newmarket Press, 18 East 48th
St., New York, NY 10017.

First Edition

10 9 8 7 6 5 4 3 2 1

Library of Congress Cataloging-in-Publication Data
Kenley, Joan.
    Whose body is it anyway? : smart choices for women / Joan Kenley, with
John C. Arpels.
        p.   cm.
    Includes index.
    ISBN 1-55704-354-X (hc)
    1. Middle aged women—Health and hygiene. I. Arpels, John C. II. Title.
    RA778.K385   1998
    613'.04244—dc21   98-11514
                                                                   CIP

Quantity Purchases
Companies, professional groups, clubs, and other organizations may
qualify for special terms when ordering quantities of this title. For information, write Special Sales, Newmarket Press, 18 East 48th Street, New
York, NY 10017, call (212) 832-3575, or fax (212) 832-3629.

Designed by Tania Garcia

Front jacket photograph by George Fry, Atherton, CA

Manufactured in the United States of America

Portions of this edition appeared previously in the author's self-published book, A Woman's
Right to Know.

For speaking engagements, seminars and workshops, contact: Dr. Joan Kenley 1-800-820-2010

THIS BOOK IS DEDICATED TO

MAGGI THRALL

1921–1992

❧

Friend, confidante, sister and second mother, who not only offered me unconditional love in all my projects, hopes and dreams, but knew how to speak generously to me about her caring in words I could hear. This was a woman who pursued a healthy life and lived with curiosity, talent and passion. She died much too early for all of us who cherished her as our angel on earth.

ADVISORY COUNCIL

Acknowledgments

First and foremost, very special thanks to two good friends and invaluable contributors: John C. Arpels, M.D., gynecologist, menopause specialist and founding member of the North American Menopause Society, has made major contributions to the information in this book as Medical Advisor and cherished colleague. His passion to help women achieve symptom relief from menopause and long-term health is an inspiration. Dr. Arpels has the capacity to micromanage each woman's treatment in a way that is unmatched; and Nancy Hicks Maynard, consultant in new media technology, journalist, lawyer, co-owner of the Oakland Tribune newspaper for ten years and treasured friend, has provided invaluable editorial expertise in the creation of this manuscript. Her talent for clarity and objectivity kept the focus. Without her support, suggestions and encouragement, this book would not have become a reality.

Also, I am especially grateful to:

The Advisory Council—John C. Arpels, Lonnie Barbach, Patricia T. Kelly, Fredi Kronenberg, Saralyn Mark, and Sherie Viencek.

Special Consultants—Risa Kagan, Anne Dosher;

The Maypole Dialogue Group—Sherrin Bennett, Sue Bethanis, Lem Bishop, Juanita Brown, Sarita Chawla, Kristin Cobble, Barbara Coffman, Anne Dosher, Andrea Dyer, Michael Exeter, Craig Fleck, Sharon Franquemont, Margaret Harris, Roger Harrison, David Isaacs, Ronita Johnson, Glenn Lehrer, Sharon Lehrer, Ken Murphy, Stephanie Ryan, Cindy Saunders, Mitch Saunders, Peggy Sebera;

Dr. Peter P. Farmer and Kathy Farmer for the use of their *Your Health Advisor and You* at the end of this book; Colleagues and friends—Ruth Owades, the Robert C. Maynard family, Katherine and Robert Franco, Suzanne Schofield, Tom Sillen, Linda Prout, Vickie Jenkins, Mary Thé, Julia Boudakian, Jon Schulberg, Bonnie Solow, Sue Cooley Ricketson, Suzie Pascal, Sally Helgesen, Michaela Cassidy, Beth Anderson, Deborah Biron, Debbie Cucalon, Maureen Deegan, Karen Hutton, Jennifer King, Paula Markovitz, Marcy Morrison, Susan Moran, Carolyn Power, Mary Ann Souza, Peg Shields, Florenzi Grant, Mary Alice Tennant, Betty Strattford,

Lucy Ramos, Lynn Newhall, Graham Simpson, Kathy Berra, Marte Pendley, David Pichette, Perry-Lynn Moffitt, Ching Chun Ou, Esther Torres, Diane Boutilier, John Lennox, Anne Sagendorph, Deborah Durga, Carole Crew, Cheryl Pombo-Soda, Diane McKallip, and Pamela St. Ives.

For assistance with the manuscript, many thanks to Mary Ann Hogan, Jamie Carroll, Sandy Rogin, Rebecca Grant, Gladys Jackson, Doreen Gray, and Leora Lee.

For helping me make this new edition of my work a reality, warm appreciation to my agents, Brooke Halpin, and Caroline Carney; editor, Keith Hollaman, and publisher, Esther Margolis.

Last, but not least, for their encouragement, support, and love, my thanks goes to Alain and Roland Gauthier; the Kiess, Spreng, Kurtz and Vorlicky families.

To anyone whom I have neglected to note here, please accept my apologies. I owe deep gratitude to so many.

CONTENTS

❧

Part II

Charts and Diagrams

FOREWORD

Welcome! It has been a privilege to be the medical advisor for Dr. Joan Kenley's book. Her friendly, conversational style of writing offers vital health information in easily understandable language. If you are trivializing your symptoms because you feel that no one, including your physician, will take you seriously, or if you think you have no choice but to accept hormone fluctuations, or if you want a private opportunity to learn about these changes, this book is for you.

In a step-by-step manner, Joan leads women through the various concerns and symptoms common to women progressing through their various health passages. It contains enough information to help you avoid awkward situations, such as having certain symptoms diagnosed as "anxiety attacks" rather than natural hormonal shifts.

You'll find helpful discussions on nutrition, sexuality, and weight issues as well as equally germane topics as the impact of stress, self-value, sleep problems, and bladder control. She also deals with three of women's biggest fears during hormonal changes—osteoporosis, heart disease, and Alzheimer's. Breast cancer, fibroids, and hysterectomy are explored in very simple, but complete, terms. One of the few authors to approach conventional and alternative treatment with balance, Dr. Kenley covers everything from the new "designer estrogens" to the Australian phytoestrogens (plant estrogens) made from red field clover. Joan is concerned with women's identity—inside and out—and includes topics not usually covered in similar health books such as self-value, cosmetic information, and plastic surgery.

A unique feature of this book is its accessible format. The print is easy to read, and important points are in bold, so readers can zero in on the most pertinent information quickly. The book is filled with charts, diagrams, and simple graphics which provide strong visual aids that are good for learning. In addition, this format encourages each reader to design her own route through the natural transitions of aging.

Women everywhere face hormone changes at some time in their life. If you haven't yet gone through menopause, some of you might have indications that this journey has begun in your early thirties, others not until your mid-forties, and some of you will sail through hormone changes without any idea of what your friends are talking about. Most of you were told that you would not experience such things as hot flashes, night sweats, or mood changes until your "menopause moment" arrived. Sorry. Many symptoms of hormone fluctuations can occur before you stop having regular periods.

Whose Body Is It Anyway? contains a very complete health picture about what women need to know. If we missed one of your issues, please write and tell us about it so we can include it in the next edition. There is no standard treatment which will work for all of you, but we hope that every one of you will discover a helpful pearl within these pages. Your search for health and vibrancy throughout life deserves to be supported. There are many options for achieving your optimal wellness. Once you discover the best choices for yourself, you will realize that a good quality of life is not a luxury—it is your right. May you enjoy reading this book as much as we enjoyed putting it together.

Best of luck,
John C. Arpels, M.D.

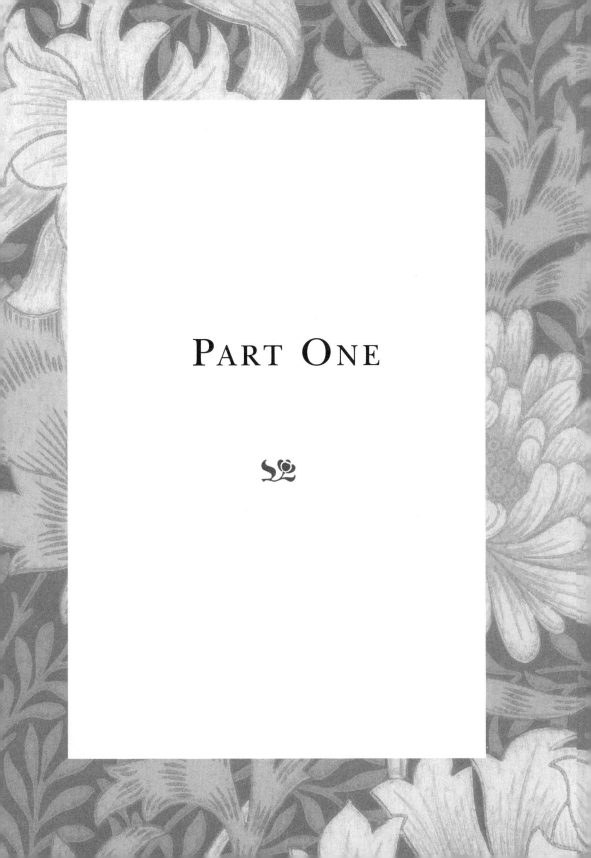

PART ONE

CHAPTER ONE

Know It, Choose It, Use It

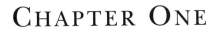

Know it — *Stop the mystery.*

Choose it — *Find your path.*

Use it — *Take action right away.*

—*Joan Kenley*

FULL MOON MORNING

It's a full moon morning
Fore the sun starts yawning
And a song is dawning in my soul

If you dwell in possibility and
Trust your inner heart to see
Maybe we could all Be Well
There's a Sacred Calling to Be Well

If you know it, choose it, use it
Then there's no chance to confuse it,
Can't you tell . . .

Know it — Stop the mystery
Choose it — Find your path
Use it — Take action right away

You'll need Love and Will and Passion
'Cause it won't be easy passin' thru these times

It's our full moon morning
Time for all women yearning to Be Well

Come with me — Learn with me — Be Well

Joan Kenley
—Dedicated to Anne

Know It, Choose It, Use It

❧

I'd like to welcome you to the health discoveries that can ignite hope for wellness in every sense of the word—mental, emotional, physical, and spiritual. For too many years, our culture has promoted the negative message that not long after age thirty our youth will wind down while the erosion of our aging will speed up. Bizarre myths about menopause are rampant. Seniorlife optimal wellness is uncharted. Confusion is at an all-time high. On the one hand, today's women appear to be experiencing change-of-life symptoms earlier than ever; on the other hand, women are breast feeding with bifocals! Women too often assume that unexpected disturbances in their mind/body/soul states are about anything except the effect of changing hormones and the natural process of growing older.

It's time to break through these dilemmas by offering you the smart choices that are available through the latest research about your ever-shifting health landscape. It's time to break through concerns that can be overwhelming and cause:

- denial that we aren't truly feeling in top form,
- doubt that anyone will be available to listen sensitively to our confusion or pain, and
- despair that the treatment options are too dangerous to embrace or trust.

By lifting the veil of misinformation and encouraging action that will lead to options you can trust, this book will help you find your own personal approach to extend any-age good health into seniorlife zest.

Having lived through a rough mid-forties transition, I searched and researched wellness answers with both desperation and optimism. After gathering mountains of information and finding various treatments that proved to be successful, I started a renewed quest to also find answers for my friends and clients. I interviewed leading experts in the field and was able to form an outstanding Advisory Council.

Janine O'Leary Cobb of Toronto, Canada, leaped into the abyss of women in need of information by publishing, in 1984, one of the first newsletters for menopausal women, *A Friend In Need*, years before the devastating wall of ignorance about midlife health began to crumble. She says, "I vividly remember coming across the printed lecture notes about menopause distributed to third year medical students: 'Well adjusted women have no problem with menopause.' Just by asking a doctor about menopause, I had labeled myself as maladjusted." Unfortunately, even today, this can still be the case.

In 1991, Gail Sheehy brought the subject of "menopause" out of the closet with *The Silent Passage*. Lila E. Nachtigall, M.D., and Joan Heilman, who authored their book *Estrogen* in the same year, revealed valuable hormone facts and detailed female health guidance to us. Not far behind came more titles that are listed in back, along with the names of a number of women's health newsletters. These periodicals can be a wonderful source of helpful, readable articles that will help keep you abreast of the latest information.

My hope is that you will use this book to personalize your health issues, because you're not just "one-in-a-million," you're "one-of-a-kind." To balance the picture, you'll find recommendations that often include both traditional and alternative (or "complementary") healing practices.

My aim is to:

- answer the questions that are on your mind
- give you easy-to-understand information
- save you time and money
- prevent heartache and confusion

What energized me to pursue more and more answers again and again were the countless personal stories that broke my heart. Does this scenario sound familiar?

> *I met Margaret, a forty-eight-year-old career woman, at a friend's house. She heard about my passion to educate women concerning their health choices, and she wanted to talk to me about her menopause dilemmas. She told me she always goes to health consultations repeating a pattern of confusion. She vows each time to change her behavior. She'll plan what to ask and what to challenge; she'll refuse to feel like a passive victim of someone else's view; she'll be informed about the treatment suggestions.*
>
> *But now that menopause is approaching, she's more confused than ever. She's not quite sure just what she needs to know from her doctor, but she does have meaningful questions.*
>
> *During the visit, Margaret is stunned to feel mentally fuzzy or even blank. She surrenders her agenda to the doctor's opinions and treatment advice, taking cues from this authority figure: "Time is short. The prescription you've been handed will take care of everything. Nothing else is needed." Margaret is not given a reading list or instructions on how to find more information or other treatment options.*
>
> *A few hours after leaving the office, she has the sinking realization that she indeed has forgotten to ask the most worrisome question. She is vaguely aware that she put her*

questions aside because she didn't want to disturb her practitioner's tight schedule or to appear foolish.

On the other hand, Margaret was not asked if she was experiencing memory problems, mild disorientation, or difficulty learning new tasks — so she wasn't confronted with the symptoms she fears most: symptoms of a very serious disease. For several months, Margaret has been secretly terrified that she might be suffering from signs of early Alzheimer's. Although no mental or physical changes should be discounted or undiagnosed, she realizes from her conversation with me that her behavior is more likely to be caused by midlife biological changes that are sometimes just temporary — such as short-term memory loss, problems with learning skills, problems focusing, or problems coping — and often can be improved with treatments and behavioral changes.

If you have a similar story to tell — or any other that makes you feel unable to take an active role in your health — this book will help. But if you agree that personal health action is a cause you choose to take on, you may have to consider yourself one of the early pioneers. What needs to shift is the current, prevailing pattern of patient behavior from uninformed and obedient to participating health partner. And if you are among those fortunates who have excellent partnering with your health advisors, you can encourage others to look for the same.

Here are some important questions to ask yourself:
- How do you think about your aches, pains, shortcomings, and illnesses?
- Do you feel that your circumstances are responsible for your well-being or ill-being? Do you suffer from self-blame?

- How do you talk to yourself about these matters? What messages do you glean from your personal reflections? What positive plans do you make?
- Do you go into denial, victim mode, anger, wishful thinking, or outreach and action?
- Do you act as if your doctor or therapeutic counselor should have all the answers? Do you choose to look for more than one option as you also inform yourself? Have you thought about what steps you could take to partner with your health practitioner or others for optimal healing?

After reflecting upon your answers to these questions, you can also consider the various dynamics of not feeling totally well or of being ill. Think about the physical, emotional, mental, and spiritual influences that can come into the picture. Look at healing from all these dimensions, even though there's no clear-cut way to determine the specific role that each one will play. But by focusing on all of these dimensions—instead of just one or two—you expand your possibilities for overall wellness. And you don't have to have a specific ailment to get your arms around how these questions can stimulate even more careful prevention and a better quality of life.

Various Dimensions of Illness

Physical: heredity, genetic makeup, aging, biological changes, injuries, fatigue, sleep deprivation, abuse of drugs and/or alcohol, smoking or second-hand smoke, eating habits, effects of child bearing, environmental causes such as toxins and radiation, etc.

Emotional: self-control, self-esteem, relationships, stress, loss, disconnection from yourself, feeling unloved, isolation, shame, and guilt.

Mental: self-criticism, pessimistic outlook, information overload, obligations, burdens, and distorted perceptions.

Spiritual: no reason for living, loss of meaning, no identification with a higher purpose, fear of death, no sense of the sacred in your life, and no connection to a higher power.

It's truly sad to report that there are certain surgeons, physicians, and nurses who don't want to be challenged by your knowledge, questions, or participation in your own wellness.

A few years ago, when I had to make six visits to several hospitals—including some emergency rooms—over a three month period, I received quite an education about the real world of hospitalization. I had naively assumed that the caregivers would welcome an informed patient but I found that this was not necessarily so. While many of my experiences were positive, some of my requests caused animosity, and the input I provided about my case was often ignored. Twice I almost died. Of course, treatment and attitudes can vary tremendously from one hospital to another and even from one day to the next in the same facility.

I discovered that the expertise of the anesthesiologist is just as important as the skill of the surgeon. There are new technologies in the field that do not leave patients nauseated, drugged, or exhausted after receiving a general anesthetic. A serious conversation before the day of surgery with whoever may be involved in putting you to sleep can prevent many unfortunate and unnecessary aftereffects.

Office visits can cause other dilemmas. A great number of women have assumed that health advisors can prescribe a course of prevention, health management, or treatment options almost magically, all in a twenty-minute visit. However, before any examination is done or tests are given, a comprehensive consultation is necessary. It must include an in-depth conversation about your personal and family health history and your current symptoms, lifestyle habits, dietary choices, and emotional or stress influences.

Most importantly, you need a compassionate, caring practitioner—someone you trust absolutely. Rachel Naomi Remen, M.D., had a cancer patient who told her, "My doctor's love is as important to me as his chemotherapy, but he does not know it." In her authentic and moving book, *Kitchen Table Wisdom,* Dr. Remen reveals, "For a long time, I had carried the belief that as a physician my love didn't matter and the only thing of value I had to offer was my knowledge and skill. My training had argued me out of my truth. Medicine is as close to love as it is to science, and its relationships matter even at the edge of life itself."

It's comforting to find health advisors who recognize the value of their roles as healers as well as technicians. For those doctors who can't or won't include the time for personal healing contact in the patient/health advisor relationship, there is an alternative to consider. Offices can offer appointments with a health advocate or nurse practitioner to take your history, answer questions, and provide quality listening. This arrangement can promote a feeling of safety and respect with the opportunity for you to bring up any concerns you have.

One of the best resources for menopausal educational materials and a list of mid- to seniorlife physicians in your area is the North American Menopause Society. You can call 1 (800) 774-5342 to receive the doctors' names and a complimentary "Menopac." Also check their website at *www.menopause.org* for other information.

Two first-rate books to know about to prepare you for doctor visits are:
- Joe and Teresa Graedon's *The People's Guide to Deadly Drug Interactions.* (Also, be sure to see the chart on page xx.)

• *Good Operations — Bad Operations* by Charles B. Inlander and the Staff of the People's Medical Society.

When you are paying attention to your emotional, mental, and physical dimensions with an educated awareness, you can contribute significant information during your health appointments. Let's face it — you can be an expert, excellent resource for your wellness because you live with yourself twenty-four hours a day. Besides, knowing your behavior and reactions on various levels can help you help yourselves in all matters, not just your health. An extremely useful commentary and questionnaire written by Peter P. Farmer, M.D., and his wife, Kathy Farmer, P.A., about getting the most from your relationship with your doctor or health advisor is included in the back of this book, and I strongly urge you to use it.

If self-awareness or self-learning hasn't already been part of your life, it's worth considering. Discovering how to become more awake about your own personal nature and the deep meaning the awareness can bring to your life can be an extraordinarily valuable pursuit. I have been fortunate to be trained in and healed by many disciplines, including mind/body psychology, the spiritual development of A.H. Almaas' Diamond Heart work, and psychotherapy with Drs. Clinton and Clifton Kew. All experiences were extremely valuable and life-changing. All encouraged the development of compassion, awareness, objectivity, and a love for the truth.

❦

Before you make any health appointments, don't forget to look over this book for subjects you feel you would like to explore further, or health options you might like to consider. You could make a copy of the Diagnostic

Questionnaire in the back of this book and mail it to your doctor in advance. You could take this book along to your visit; use it both as a reminder and as an aid in communicating your questions and expressing interest in selecting your own treatment choices.

It's a smart idea to record your office conversations for later review. The emotion of the moment can cause you to misinterpret — or possibly miss altogether — some very important points. Review your notes and play the tape after you come home while the visit is still fresh in your mind. And if your appointment is about a serious health matter, taking a family member or health advocate with you can provide tremendous personal support.

With this pep talk in mind, when you take on the role of an inspired, health-active woman: do it boldly. Shout it. Even sing it. My lyrics are:

> KNOW IT ——— *Stop the mystery.*
> CHOOSE IT ——— *Find your path.*
> USE IT ——— *Take action right away.*

These words are designed with a serious purpose. Take note of the sobering information that was conveyed in the educational publication *Menopause Management,* endorsed by the North American Menopause Society. The research confirms that:

- Few women know what prevention, health, menopause, and seniorlife information they need.
- The resulting confusion makes choices difficult.
- Many of those who are given courses of treatment, exercise plans, behavioral changes, or food modification don't use — or follow through with — the suggestions given by the health practitioner.

Realizing how painfully true this reality is worked on me and in me as I wrote about what I felt women needed in order to take action. Over the years of my experience with the clients in my consulting practice as well as in my circle of female friends, I witnessed the same pattern over and over again. Caring, well-meaning women are more likely to see that their husbands, children, siblings, and parents get to the doctor long before they schedule any visits for themselves for checkups, chronic symptoms, or specific illnesses. Would my book motivate these same women to behave differently? Chances were that it would not, based on education, information, and pep-talks alone. That's when I came up with the idea that would appeal to the womanly caregiver and promote her role as care-receiver in return.

THE PROMISE BETWEEN FRIENDS

The following contract is a commitment between two friends for one year to help each other schedule important regular checkups and, if needed, offer companionship through illness, hospital visits, and emotionally charged health appointments. Please, seriously consider inviting one of your friends to enter into this agreement with you.

If any part of the Promise feels uncomfortable, just cross it out.

Promise Between Friends Contract

As of this date, _____, I promise for one year to remind you about each health check-up that is recommended for your health history and age and, if you want me to, I will go along with you for support. You will, in turn, promise the same help for me. When possible, we will try to schedule the same kind of appointments on the same day, even if not in the same office — mammograms, physicals, blood tests, OB-GYN exams, and other health visits.

When we have each listened fully to the other's point of view, I won't argue with you or blame you for any treatment decisions you care to make

We agree to share honestly any helpful, non-judgmental observations that may encourage each of us to achieve a more healthful quality of life.

We will stand by one another, knowing that any treatment or lifestyle choice can bring up resistance to long-term follow-through.

When compassion and self-love seem to be absent, we will remember to invite those feelings to re-emerge.

Each of us will find the right match if we don't already have physicians or care providers that we absolutely love and trust.

We commit to tell the full truth about our health behavior and treatment practices as well as to reveal all therapies to each of our doctors and health advisors.

We pledge not to feel guilty about any physical or emotional trials that come our way and will not blame ourselves for any illnesses or other life challenges.

If we both find it comfortable, we will share our dark thoughts, current concerns, and worries regarding possible future problems — emotional, physical, and spiritual — along with the dreams and wishes we have for ourselves and others.

Should either of us be faced with a serious or life-threatening illness, we promise to have open conversations about all our hopes and fears about death and dying.

Your friend in health,

_____

Now and in the future, consider that an ounce of good prevention or appropriate care to improve the quality of your life is worth more than I can say. Join me and millions of other women on the road to self-health discovery. Find out just why these important years can be the most satisfying, sensual, sensational time of all.

Think of your life as a special kind of journey. Consider this guidebook your personal map. Remember, growing into maturity with grace and radiance is an art. Preparing for a long and healthy life has countless rewards.

Midlife isn't an ending — it's a beginning.

Menopause isn't a disease to cure, a flaw to deny, a condition to be reversed. It's an awakening.

MIDLIFE IS A GATEWAY TO HONOR.

SENIORLIFE IS AN ACCOMPLISHMENT TO REVERE.

"Whether in midlife or seniorlife, now is the time. The smart choices come only in you and through you — you can author your wellness. Make the rest of your life the best of your life."

— Joan Kenley

CHAPTER TWO

Taking a Stand:
My Own Story

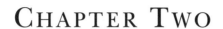

"An invitation to care givers

from every woman:

See me.

Hear me.

Know me."

—Joan Kenley

Taking a Stand: My Own Story

❧

*I*n my early forties, I earned a Ph.D. in psychology while working full time in broadcasting and coaching clients how to improve the sound of their speaking voice, years before personal vocal problems had led me to pioneer my own method of vocal improvement. I later explored this subject from the added perspectives of emotional understanding, physical/mental/spiritual awareness, and overall human development.

My first book, *Voice Power — A Breakthrough Method to Improve Your Speaking Voice,* was first published in the late eighties by Dodd Mead and Henry Holt & Company. Many of the clients who contributed to that material were important for the creation of *Whose Body Is It Anyway?* Because wellness is important for optimal vocal enhancement, my voice coaching always included conversations about health choices.

I began to hear from my female clients how their general complaints and specific mental/physical symptoms weren't taken seriously by many physicians, and how the health connection with their emotional and spiritual well-being was almost totally ignored. Here was a pattern that I felt must be changed. I believed that if women were given an opportunity to learn the information concerning the bigger picture of woman-health, the situation could improve. Couldn't practitioners learn to meet this larger scope of wellness? Then, unexpectedly, I was faced with my own health challenges.

At age forty-five, I began to ask gynecologists what to expect of menopause. As each year passed, I wondered with curiosity how my body was progressing toward this particular life transition. I was told that I'd know "it" when it happened. But I knew "it" couldn't happen overnight. In fact, some rather mild but unpleasant physical symptoms were already occurring that I couldn't explain based on my scanty information. No one was talking about this subject and the books and newsletters that are easily available now didn't exist.

During this time I was married for the first time to a charming, dynamic French leadership consultant, Alain Gauthier. I also became second mother to his talented, lovable son, Roland.

Although immensely happy with my new home and family life at age fifty, I battled with a loss of interest in other parts of my life. Trying to ignore my increasing lack of vitality, I focused on remodeling our home and grounds with a singleness of purpose. I made demoralizing attempts to manage both my mental and physical difficulties before I discovered I was suffering from several debilitating menopausal symptoms — hormone depletion, sleep deprivation, and high cholesterol.

To add to these problems, yet another burden: I had been plagued by a lifetime of weight gain and loss, but had been doing fairly well until I gained more weight than ever during those years leading to menopause. I felt trapped and angry — tangled in a mystery story with no one to track down the suspects. Here I was, exercising with trainers three to four times a week, following a limited-calorie, healthy, very low fat food regime, and gaining weight. I couldn't stabilize or lose. Digging into my worn-out will in an effort to be healthy and to shed those pounds, I over-exercised, causing physical exhaustion that took me weeks to recover from. I was bewildered. I felt betrayed by my own body. Fortunately, through much research and determination, I found a solution to the weight I had gained and eventually improved my workout stamina. Treatment for my symptoms began to take hold.

Then, for nine months, I had intermittent heavy menopausal bleeding that left me energetically compromised and anemic. I needed help. I scheduled a visit for a natural progesterone injection to stop the bleeding and a B12 injection to boost my energy. To save time, I went to a doctor I had not met before. The internist first began by challenging the prescription strength my gynecologist had called in for the progesterone injection. He showed no concern that I had been bleeding for three weeks and was so exhausted I found it difficult to speak.

Then, out of the blue, he was shouting at me, saying that administering the vitamin shot would be unethical, even though it had been helpful to me and many of my colleagues in the past. After abusing me with this tirade, this tall, imperious physician told me he wasn't interested in patients self-diagnosing their conditions. He proceeded to slam the door behind him as he made a grand exit, leaving me to sob uncontrollably. I felt grateful when the nurse practitioner offered to take over from there, but only to administer the progesterone shot.

After some research, I was determined to solve my problem without rushing into a hysterectomy. I decided to have an endometrial ablation, an out-patient laser procedure, to burn away the lining of the uterus. This was to eliminate the endometrium build-up that was diagnosed as causing the heavy bleeding episodes, even though the ultrasound pictures did not indicate any abnormalities in my uterus.

Knowing that nausea could be a big discomfort with general anesthesia, I chose a month in advance to have an epidural injection in my spine that would block the pain and allow me to stay awake and view the surgery on a video screen. As I was being prepped, the anesthesiologist breezed in, asking what we were up to, without having consulted my surgeon in advance about my specific preferences. I explained my request and he carried on and on about the chance that an epidural might give me such an untreatable headache afterward that I might suffer without relief for a week. Believe me, I had no room on my calendar for seven days of this kind of excruciating pain, but I had no one to consult and I was under the influence of a brain functioning in extreme slow-motion.

Then, he refused to administer anti-nausea medication during the procedure, telling me he always did that post-surgery, which I knew would not work for me. That blew it. Here I was, a woman who does not break down easily, sobbing for an hour before I went into surgery, with nurses encouraging me to reschedule. I resolved to tough it out. Result: I did have the epidural, and the nausea lasted for six hours afterward. Those extra hours before the hospital would release me cost $600. The possible "incurable" week-long headache did not surface. Later, I learned that there is a simple, fast-acting remedy if a post-epidural headache occurs. You can imagine my reaction.

A week later, like a faucet being turned on without warning, blood cascaded down my legs while standing in a shop with a friend I was visiting in Oregon. This was not the "spotting" the surgeon had mentioned, in passing, that might happen from time to time. I was shocked and scared, but when my surgeon was reached, he claimed it was perfectly "normal." I knew it was not. It would have been even more frightening if I could have known what was in store for me in the next few months.

More short episodes of this faucet-like bleeding, with the addition of large clots, occurred upon my return from Oregon. A few days later, while I was being filmed in my home for a major network television interview, I had to excuse myself several times because the hemorrhaging was too much for my "Super Diapers," ordinarily used for incontinence. I began to forget what each question was halfway through the answer. The producer and crew were angels, offering plenty of chances to answer or to fly in again if that was going to be better for me. Having gotten "gussied up" for the session, I was determined to see it through, and did. But as soon as the interview was over, my husband rushed me to the hospital for another surgical procedure.

The next weekend while I was at home recovering, I lost half my blood volume. My husband was not able to reach my surgeon or anyone in his office who was willing to advise us about where to go or whom to see. The emergency room at a nearby hospital told us to call an ambulance and get there as quickly as possible. After two days of transfusions and drug therapy, I flew half-way across the country, requiring the use of airport wheelchairs and a supportive companion to accompany me, so I could fulfill an assignment to deliver a speech for three thousand people.

Looking back, this seems truly absurd. Obviously, my powers of decision making were distorted. Meeting these obligations was a silly way of convincing myself that I was really okay. After all, my surgeon didn't find any cause for alarm when I told him about the emergency room incident. He told me I should simply stay home for a week with a rather uncomfortable catheter in my uterus, which should certainly heal whatever problem I had been having. Great. Anything to stop this mess. Since I had sometimes felt fairly well between episodes, I kept thinking that all this probably wasn't such big a deal. But it was a big deal.

With the "catheter week" behind me and no problems for a few weeks, expectations of no more trouble ran high. I trustingly saw my husband off to France and waved good-bye to my son who was going to be away for the holiday weekend. I was looking forward to a nice quiet Thanksgiving, resting and reading in bed.

As this lovely Thursday began, I was feeling physically well and took time to focus gratefully on those who had kept me going over the years and particularly during these major difficulties: Sherie Viencek, D.C., with her chiropractic and coping treatments; Betty Strattford, M.D., with homeopathic remedies; Dr. Julia Boudakian with cranial-sacral therapy; and Dr. Chin Chun Ou, with acupuncture — all talented, outstanding Bay Area practitioners and healers with compassion and perceptions beyond any methodology that can be easily described. While in this reverie of thankfulness, I suspected I was starting to bleed again and tried hard to wish it away.

When I finally had to acknowledge this first moderate hemorrhage, I slowly cleaned up the bathroom and decided to be very still and just stay in bed quietly with my feet up praying for no more trouble. I wasn't worried. Not even after the second one. After the third, I began to be concerned, but desperately hoped I wouldn't have to call an ambulance on a holiday and go once again through another emergency room experience. I began to get cold and was especially glad I had lit a fire in the fireplace earlier. I went from blind denial to horrified disbelief when I had yet another hemorrhage — how could I be losing so much blood in so few hours? Then I began to get dizzy and lightheaded. Reluctantly I called one of my nearby friends, all the time thinking I didn't want to bother anyone, especially on Thanksgiving. No one answered.

Muddled as I had become, I knew I no longer had any choice. I had to call the ambulance. It was difficult to pronounce the words just to tell the 911 operator where I was. I passed out and then heard yelling outside. The paramedics had arrived but the doors were locked. They were shouting and knocking loudly, but I had no voice to answer and I was not sure I could make it to the door. I crawled, passed out, crawled again. Even then I couldn't help thinking this was worse than a B-movie as I reached up from the floor to turn the knob just before they started to axe down the entryway. In no time I was on oxygen and in the ambulance.

The emergency room was literally both a lifesaver and a place from hell. Once my vital signs were stabilized, I realized I was in a lot of pain. Nevertheless, I was carted off to the side of a large dark room with needles and drips. No one who passed would respond to my questions or my discomfort. When a nurse or intern would come by to check on me, that's all they would do — check. No answers. No information. Finally I was told I would be put in a room when they found one available. I'd been there for three hours when my good friend arrived with comfort and a hand to hold in that cold-hearted room. When she left after 11 p.m., neither of us thought it would take until 2:30 a.m. for me to be taken to a room and a bed. My good luck was to have the most cheerful, helpful nurse anyone could wish for to get me settled and to sleep.

At this point I was adamant about scheduling myself for a hysterectomy. Who could I trust? What hospital should I choose? I was not going to die to save my uterus. The very kind gynecologist in charge at this trauma center spent over an hour with me the next day going over my case. He offered to locate a surgeon who would perform the hysterectomy in the hospital of my choice and to return my phone calls if I needed help in the meantime. He came through in every way.

When I checked into the last hospital for my final surgery, I chose to try to curtail any possible difficulties by filling out the "complaint form" as if it were a "request form" the day before I checked in. I asked for a long discussion with the anesthesiologist so I wouldn't suffer from nausea after the surgery. Dr. Joseph Bermudez not only talked to me at length, but he performed an epidural anesthesia with perfection and with a kindness of spirit. I had no nausea after-effects. I requested nurses with compassion and an ability to listen, and each one was top-notch. I had no worries about Dr. Edward Blumenstock, my sensitive and brilliant surgeon. Every phase went smoothly, contrary to some of my earlier experiences with other, but not all, physicians, caregivers, and hospitals.

Only after the surgery was the real cause of the difficulty discovered by the pathologist: exposed blood vessels in the neck of the cervix, an extremely rare occurrence, but not unheard of. It is not something that can be diagnosed with current imaging techniques.

Today I am enjoying a wonderful new lease on life, bursting with passion to share with women everywhere the health messages I have gathered for this book.

"In the shadow of illness,

Wellness beckons;

The flame of courage

flickers;

And our trust in the

Universe is

all that it is."

—Joan Kenley

CHAPTER THREE

Briefly— The Basics

"In the seasons of life, thrashing through the denial, the mystery, the innocence, and the ignorance of our body changes is always more painful than standing in the middle of truth."

—*Joan Kenley*

BRIEFLY—THE BASICS

❧

*T*his chapter gives a brief survey of very basic information, answering the questions women ask most about:

• specific health changes,
• hormone dilemmas,
• menopause concerns, and
• wellness after fifty.

Remarkably, certain female health concerns continue to be "secret subjects," even in this day and age. Myths and outdated beliefs cloud the issues. Unverified, grossly incorrect information takes hold with repetition, even when there is no basis in truth.

The information here is not just for women who are thirty-five to fifty-five, but also for the post-menopausal and seniorlife woman. Much of the current information wasn't known in the not-too-distant past. Significant biological changes which occur at midlife contribute to so many later unfortunate conditions, many of which are preventable.

Jane Brody tells us in *Jane Brody's Nutrition Book,* "I believe that people are most likely to loosen their hold on old habits and make constructive changes in their lives when they understand and appreciate the rationale for those changes and are given some guidance as to how to go about them." This philosophy reflects the intention of *Whose Body Is It Anyway?*

STANDARD TREATMENTS, ALTERNATIVE THERAPIES, PLACEBO EFFECT, AND TRUST

There are four major considerations I would suggest for you to take into account when making decisions concerning your health care.

"Standard," "conventional," "orthodox," and "traditional" are all terms used to refer to Western medicine that are commonly used throughout this country to treat countless conditions. They include the treatments of acute diseases and surgical procedures. Doctors with medical degrees in the United States are generally "allopathic" physicians, a term used to indicate graduates of medical schools practicing "conventional" medicine.

Alternative/complementary therapies are mentioned throughout this book as treatment choices. You'll find definitions of many alternative/complementary healing practices in the back of this book in the "Alternative/Complementary Glossary." A majority of these methods are about keeping you well, balancing your mind/body system, easing or curing chronic conditions, and/or reducing pain and enhancing structural problems. The guiding purpose of these systems is to treat causes, not just symptoms. Almost half of all patients in this country seek some form of non-traditional treatment.

The placebo effect involves the positive conscious or unconscious belief in your treatment choice, which can greatly affect the results of any regimen and, as we know, can make even sugar pills powerful. It is reported that the placebo factor in any regimen can be as high as 30 to 40 percent!

Trust in an empowering, partnering relationship with your healthcare advisor can enhance your overall health situation tremendously. It can strengthen your peace of mind to remember that you can always change treatment directions — without a moment of guilt — any time you feel the occasion calls for it. And if you have more than one health practitioner, tell each one about the other(s). Any embarrassment you may have about loyalties to more than one doctor, counselor, or treatment only undermines everyone involved and may be extremely harmful to you.

Alternative therapies can be incorporated into standard medical practices or they can serve as the primary treatment for various illnesses. When dealing with serious health concerns, you have to choose for yourself — using reliable information — which discipline will best serve your healing as well as inspire your faith and confidence. When appropriate, you might consider a combination of disciplines rather than an either/or approach.

The subjects you'll encounter in this chapter will provide brief information about some of women's major concerns: emotional dismay, bone disease, hormone concerns, sleep problems, hot flashes, Pap smears, lovemaking, hysterectomy, and more. Later chapters will have detailed material on these topics and many others.

This is only the beginning.

❧

MEMORY AND PROBLEM SOLVING

Does your brain ever feel like Teflon? Do matters that were always easy to recall float into some strange mist? Have you found yourself suffering from what might be called a "decision-making disorder"? Have you been unexpectedly caught in the middle of a "dysfunction junction" during a perfectly ordinary situation?

Do you ever ask yourself, "Where did I leave my keys? Where did I park my car? Is the dentist appointment Tuesday or Thursday? What's the name of that store?" If so, you might think you're coming down with premature senility. But don't panic if you feel like you're trying to cope with a wavy, gravy brain. You're probably just having manageable short-term memory glitches or foggy mental functions that come with hormone changes and aging. Nouns and names can be harder to recall — you can humorously refer to it as "noun-itis." For a few years you may need to adopt an abundant use of "that thing," "you know, that person," and "it's that whatyamacallit." You're not losing your marbles, but you may be losing your recall. Also, you may be trying to keep track of too many things.

If declining estrogen levels are depleting the reserves in your short-term memory bank, consider this: the places in your brain that store new information may not be getting their "minimum daily requirement" of estrogen, so they may slightly misfire. The result: "Where in the world is my purse?" "Just what did I come into this room to find?"

Decreased oxygen to the brain as we age can also play a significant role in memory and brain function. This gives us yet another important reason for including heart-activating, oxygen-pumping exercise in our health plans.

However, don't ignore the fact that memory problems can have other causes. Chronic fatigue syndrome (CFS), for instance, can influence memory and mental acuity. So can stress, depression, and fatigue. If symptoms indicate further exploration, it's wise to get a complete professional diagnosis. But don't worry. Statistically, the chance that you may be experiencing early signs of Alzheimer's Disease is very slim.

Homeopathy, acupuncture, phytoestrogen supplements, and certain nutritional regimens such as gingko bilboa can improve or remove these memory difficulties. Estrogen replacement therapies that are totally or predominately formulated with 17B estradiol (Estrace®) seem to be slightly more efficient for memory problems than esterified equine estrogens (Premarin® and Estratab®). See Chapter Four for more information.

There was an embroidered pillow I saw in a mail order catalogue that struck my fancy. It said, "I've got it all together, but I forgot where I put it!"

It's possible that after menopause your memory can be better than ever. In the meantime, write things down. Carry your notebook with you. Set timers or mini-wrist alarms for reminders. Send yourself voice mail or e-mail messages. Tuck a small tape recorder in your purse. Above all, don't volunteer to be a memory bank for anyone else's deposits.

BONE CONCERNS AND OSTEOPOROSIS

Osteoporosis is often called "the brittle bone disease" and it can develop silently over many years. Some thirty-something women may already have it without knowing it. At the same time, women in their thirties and forties also can take steps to prevent suffering from it later. Loss of height, a curved spine, or a "dowager's hump" can result from this bone condition. These spinal changes in turn can put pressure on the diaphragm that can cause difficulty in breathing, as well as compression of all the abdominal organs. Each year, many women with osteoporosis lose their independence by fracturing a hip or a vertebra. Death can occur from complications of hip fractures.

Women who tend to be at higher risk than others are: Asian; of Northern European origin — white, thin, and blonde; smokers; those whose periods have ceased; those with eating disorders; and non-exercisers. For a more complete list of risk factors, see Chapter Seven.

The loss of estrogen during the first few years after surgical removal of the ovaries or natural menopause can dramatically accelerate bone loss. Osteoporosis can be arrested, slowed down and, in many cases, prevented altogether. It is treatable at any age. Find out more by reading Chapter Four. It will tell you how weight-bearing exercise, calcium supplements, hormone replacement therapy, a calcium-rich diet, and some new non-hormonal treatments can make a very big difference.

SLEEP PROBLEMS AND ENERGY SPURTS

Health problems, emotional turmoil, and life circumstances can influence your sleep and energy tremendously. Several contributing factors may be at work.

Life's pressures can deplete estrogen levels as well as the ability to relax and sleep deeply. Similarly, hormone variations in your biological landscape can offer periodic "Super Woman" surges or huge energy drops — no energy, no staying power, no oomph. These symptoms could mean you're experiencing the hormone fluctuations that cause waking up during the night from warm waves, hot flashes, or night sweats. Maybe you're having troubled sleep because you're stressed. Or are you stressed because you're not sleeping? It's hard to tell where one cause ends and the next begins.

Consider the sections in Chapter Two concerning various therapy options. With this information in mind, see a health advisor to check for the particular source of your difficulties. Finding out how to get a good night's sleep can often be the most healing potion of all.

MOOD SWINGS

Women who overflow with joy one minute and break into tears the next need to discover why. Is there no apparent reason? Do those you love raise their eyebrows or start avoiding you? Do you wonder, "Will I ever be me again?" This roller coaster is common for women experiencing hormonal changes. However, you should bear in mind the fact that unidentified emotional shifts can result from illness, reactions to medications, and undiagnosed physical/emotional ailments.

Assuming that there are no other causes and you're truly menopausal, your hormones can be mixing up in new ways, causing the brain centers involved with emotions to behave in ways you might never have imagined. An unexpected positive or negative feeling — a big one, a strong one — can come out of left field and knock you over. At the same time, you may be experiencing changing interests, dissolving partnerships, shifting values, friends moving, children leaving, and parents dying.

Some changes are comfortable; some are painful. Even though every personality, every life change, every menopause is different, it all tends to even out with treatment, time, or a combination of both. So address any emotional passages with patience and professional advice. Cherish your challenges. Changing situations can lead you to new beginnings. Remember: this new phase can hold untold promise, power, and productivity. You're in good company. Millions of women are sharing these transitions with you.

URINARY FREQUENCY AND INCONTINENCE

Urinary difficulties often go untreated because so few women speak of them to their doctors or realize that there are various remedies that can help tremendously or even cure completely. Internal structural changes or other conditions may be involved, and you should find out. If the problem develops into incontinence, don't be embarrassed to discuss this condition with your health practitioner.

Let's face it—a frequent urgency to urinate doesn't help during any part of your twenty-four hour schedule. It's truly inconvenient no matter how you look at it. Physical changes in your urinary system might be the reason. Causes can include childbearing, hormone changes, muscle weakness, and other medical problems.

When estrogen levels drop or are depleted, the bladder and urinary tract tissue can often become thinner, drier, less elastic, and more easily irritated. Urinary tract infections (UTIs) can play a role in this problem, and these infections can increase in frequency during menopause and after, as can various causes and kinds of urinary urgency and incontinence. There are treatments, exercises, and surgical procedures available that can help relieve or eliminate these problems. This subject is addressed in detail in Chapter Five.

HOT FLASHES AND SWEATS

It can strike like lightning. It can feel like an electrical surge or a sauna or both at once. You're hot, you're clammy. You're red, you're sweating. You're having a hot flash.

A friendlier term women are using for hot flashes is "power surge." Here's what's going on: Because your hormones are out of balance, something seems to short-circuit in the brain's internal thermostat. Blood vessels constrict unpredictably. The skin temperature rises slightly. The strange part is that nobody is exactly sure why. What they do know is that hot flash "triggers" include stress, caffeine, alcohol, spicy foods, warm rooms, and nightclothes made of synthetic fabrics. Will the flashes irritate you? Maybe. Embarrass you? Only if you let them. Go away? Eventually. Want relief? See the suggestions in Chapter Five.

HEART RATE CHANGES AND CHEST PAINS

A rapidly beating or pounding heart is scary. If you're having other menopausal symptoms as well, though, chances are your heart symptoms are menopause-related; scary, but not dangerous. These palpitations are probably temporary spasms in the blood vessels that feed the heart, caused by a rapid drop or fluctuation in hormone levels. Stress, caffeine, tobacco, and even chocolate can also make your heart feel jittery. No matter how brief an episode you experience, a fluttering heart can frighten you, which in itself can lead to a change in pulse or blood pressure.

On the other hand, if symptoms persist, absolutely get a diagnosis. Just be aware that women with heart disease are frequently misdiagnosed because women's complaints differ from men's. Most heart studies have been conducted with the male population, and physicians tend to be influenced by the outdated theory that serious heart disease belongs to the male sex. This is not true. Always talk over all symptoms with your doctor. The older you are, the greater your chances for heart disease. Remember: nothing can take the place of yearly tests to check for early signs of any cardiovascular problems. And never forget that half

a million women a year die of heart disease or stroke—
many more than from any other cause.

LOVEMAKING, LOVING OTHERS, SELF-LOVE

Let's look at each aspect of the concerns which come
hand in hand with nearly every form of partnership. First,
your intimate love relationship. Just when you thought
you were headed for years of worry-free lovemaking and
more time to share with your love partner, you're faced
with some unexpected boomerangs. Your usual responses
can be filled with surprises. Having sex can seem more
exciting, suddenly uninteresting, or it may even cause
some pain. Just know there are reasons and remedies,
helpful tips, and treatments covered in Chapter Three.
Above all, don't give up on the possibility of a lifetime of
loving closeness.

Unexpected emotional feelings can be attributed to
shifting hormones, health problems, or other challenges
that have appeared at this particular time in your life. The
love you feel for friends, family, career, and other activities
can go through some rocky periods. These new emotions
can also be related to your changing values and your personal sense of worth. This behavior can be unsettling, particularly when you are going through midlife biological
transitions that can cause you to become more fragile and
more short-tempered. If you're used to feeling like a
woman of steel, you may be faced with unexpected sensations that resemble something more like crumpled tin foil
from time to time.

Be aware that there's usually an opportunity to create a
positive attitude or a negative cesspool when life changes
knock on your door, no matter what age you are. However,

if you've been holding certain feelings back for most of your life, no matter what age you are now, this can become the time when many unsaid, unfelt feelings will begin to form, float up, and emerge, finally ready to be revealed.

Often it's good to talk to other women who are going through this too, either informally or through support groups. You might seek out a professional counselor who specializes in women's issues, or talk to a health advisor who can diagnose what medications, treatments, or supplements might help to smooth things out. When you're feeling emotional or physical discomfort, it can be difficult to identify what your true feelings are. Explore with fresh eyes. Be curious. Be interested. Learn from this time of change. Focusing on the small wonderful events that live at the fingertips of our lives can plug us into gratitude just when we need it.

Self-love is probably the most difficult human quality to master and is an ever on-going process. Chances are you've felt and thought negative things about yourself in the past. Perhaps you're feeling that way now. You may think only you have this problem. Nevertheless, some degree of self-doubt and self-dislike is a trait that you have in common with most other people in the world.

This book is full of positive suggestions that can nurture the self-love process. Know that personal negativity may possibly be healed with some self-development/spiritual practice skills in hand. Know that a positive inner dialogue creates a powerful internal space. Know that self-love is always ready to take center stage, but it has to be invited.

WHAT IS MENOPAUSE?

When you think about menopause — literally defined as your last natural menstrual period — you might think it should be called menostop. However, with five to fifteen years of gradual hormonal change before menopause, some three years or more to go through it, and other possible continuing symptoms after, it certainly can't be called a "stop" or tagged as a specific moment in time. It's really a transition. It usually happens between ages forty-five and fifty-five, but it can be a thirties event as well. Women are sort of like snowflakes — no two are alike.

Heredity, diet, tobacco and alcohol intake, body type, illnesses, surgical procedures, and even where you live can play a role in determining the age at which you enter menopause. Menopause also marks a time when health and emotional concerns need to be addressed so you can learn to lead a healthy and long life.

Terms to recognize: The climacteric designates a woman's transition from her childbearing years to her non-childbearing life and a period of time after, covering ages thirty-five to sixty-five. The early climacteric is between thirty-five and forty-five; the perimenopause climacteric indicates the years just before and after menstruation ceases, between forty-five to fifty-five; and the late climacteric refers to those that are in the fifty-five to sixty-five range.

With the removal of your uterus, your periods will stop, but the hormone production of your ovaries will not. However, if both ovaries are removed, what's known as "surgical menopause" occurs right away, no matter what your age. If you have no surgeries or other medical exceptions, when will menopause happen to you? It depends on the factors already mentioned. If you're the average textbook example, it will occur at age fifty-one, with symptoms lasting two to three and a half years on average. A number of women will have symptoms for five to ten years.

MENOPAUSE SIGNS AND SYMPTOMS

Knowledge is not only power, but also a source of comfort when unexpected symptoms occur before, during, and after menopause. Being in the know helps each woman understand how hormonal transitions affect the mind, body, and spirit. As menopause approaches, less and less estrogen is produced by the ovaries, not always resulting in obvious symptoms for everyone. Estrogen is tied to hundreds of natural body functions — not only sexuality and childbearing but also memory, emotions, body temperature, sleep, and much more. Older women need to be conscious of how estrogen depletion in later years affects heart disease and osteoporosis. A quote from Dr. M. Metka of the University of Vienna is thought-provoking: "Ninety-five percent of what estrogen does is outside the female pelvis." And as Dr. Freda Lewis Hall, Director of Eli Lilly's Center for Women's Health, says, "We have to look at menopause beyond the hot flash!"

Estrogen changes can contribute to getting headaches or finally becoming free of them. If headaches plague you, the best up-to-date advice is in the recent book, *Headache Relief for Women,* by Alan M. Rapoport, M.D. and Fred D. Sheftell, M.D.

Normal symptoms of menopause can vary. You might have trouble sleeping or concentrating or remembering things. You might feel anxious or start flying off the handle for no reason. You might feel waves of heat, possibly followed by sweating and then chills—all part of the famous hot flash experience. These physical/emotional changes can feel very unnerving, but they aren't dangerous to your health. Your periods could be there one month, not there the next. Maybe heavier, maybe lighter. All are indications that your natural cycles are winding down, if no other reasons exist for these symptoms.

Sexual intercourse might become painful. Mini hot flashes can cause stomach upset. Your skin may itch, tingle, or feel "crawly." You may be nauseated because your eyesight is changing and you need vision correction.

There's no crystal ball telling which women will be affected by which symptoms. Genetics, general health, and lifestyle are significant contributors to the effects of midlife changes. Some evidence suggests that women with histories of PMS or serious post-partum blues have a more difficult time. There are women who are diagnosed as having chronic fatigue syndrome or fibromyalgia when they are exhibiting symptoms of early menopause. The reverse is true as well. There are opinions that say women with more fat cells tend to have fewer and less severe symptoms than those who are thin, but certainly this is not universally true.

As estrogen levels drop, the body naturally reacts. Eighty-five percent of American women have one or more of the menopausal symptoms mentioned here. For some there are no unpleasant experiences—periods will just end. For others it will almost feel like withdrawing from a drug. Just be clear that there are dozens of remedies and things to do that will help, from hormone replacement to homeopathic remedies, from the right kind of exercise and diet to acupuncture, ginseng, don quai root products, and many more suggestions that will be mentioned throughout this book. Check regularly with your health advisors for other ideas or recommendations. Read women's health and menopause newsletters about the latest developments—many are listed in the "Resources" section at the end of this book.

When your ovaries have finished their reproductive years

and people ask you pointed questions related to this subject, answer any way you please. I like the assured, spontaneous response Lauren Hutton laughingly proclaimed on "The Tonight Show" when asked if she planned to have children: "Not likely—I'm out of eggs!" Most importantly: even with no menopausal symptoms, aging continues. This is a time of life when more serious illness can develop. Conscious prevention becomes an extremely important matter.

PAP SMEARS

Facts about Pap smears are important because there is some confusion about the role they play in diagnosing the health of reproductive organs. Although frequently described as a test for cancer of the uterus and cervix, Pap smears are reliable only for detecting cancer of the cervix and upper vaginal cellular abnormalities. If you have monthly menstruation, the best time to have a Pap smear is two weeks after the first day of the last period.

Ovarian cancer cannot be identified with a Pap smear. There are no exact early warning signals. Family history and symptoms of swelling, bloating, indigestion, nausea, weight loss, or discomfort in the lower abdomen can be clues regarding cancer of the ovaries. To determine uterine cancer, investigate the pre-biopsy sonohysterogram and the new visually directed biopsy if any abnormal uterine cells need to be examined. The CA-125 test is not considered to be reliable.

FIBROIDS

Fibroid tumors are benign muscle growths that may cause heavy or abnormal bleeding. There are three growth patterns: within the uterine walls (most common), on the outer walls of the uterus, and under the uterine lining and into the uterine cavity. They are quite common — 40 percent of all women have these tumors, and most are not bothered by them. There are more cases of this condition among African American women than among Caucasian women.

Contrary to popular belief, fibroids hardly ever become cancerous. To assume that a rapidly growing fibroid is an indication that the tumor is not benign is frighteningly incorrect.

When a fibroid is smaller than a softball or grapefruit, it doesn't usually cause discomfort or pain. However, at any size, one or more fibroids can be the reason for heavy uterine bleeding which can cause anemia along with very uncomfortable days and nights.

What about hormone replacement therapy (HRT) and fibroids? Some women are told they would have to have their fibroids removed to be able to embark on an HRT program. Another myth. Replacement hormones do not seem to cause fibroid tumors to grow.

If you have growing fibroids and no signs of discomfort, the basic rule to follow is to have your gynecologist keep watchful attention on the situation by checking you at least every six months or as soon as any symptoms warrant an office visit.

When major discomfort and heavy bleeding cause serious quality of life problems, procedures are available to either cut off the blood supply to the fibroids, causing them to shrink, or to remove the fibroids without removing the uterus. Submucous Myomectomy as Reproductive Therapy (SMART) — a new office procedure — is designed to precisely remove fibroids vaginally to help restore or maintain fertility for women who still want to conceive.

HYSTERECTOMY

First of all, the word "hysterectomy" is misused all the time. Let us first define the procedures the term frequently covers before going further:

- hysterectomy: surgical removal of uterus only
   a) vaginal hysterectomy: vaginal removal
   b) abdominal hysterectomy: abdominal removal
- total hysterectomy: removal of uterus and cervix
- oophorectomy: removal of an ovary or ovaries

Unfortunately, there is no single word for the removal of both the uterus and ovaries—and it would be useful to have one! Surveys show that even physicians use the term hysterectomy to describe both procedures. No wonder there are women who don't know what their surgeries have removed or not removed. That knowledge alone can significantly affect your overall health and treatment choices.

Conditions that can cause a need for hysterectomy include endometriosis, prolapsed uterus, anemia, cancer, and unexplained severe pain or heavy bleeding.

If you're told by doctors or friends that "you have nothing to worry about" after any type of hysterectomy, think again. It would be preferable to adopt an attitude of becoming consciously informed rather than to assume all your problems have "gone away." You may have emotional reactions or physical complications. If you are premenopausal at the time of surgical removal of both ovaries, your body will react—with or without noticeable symptoms—to instant menopause. You may have some of the menopausal health or behavior aftereffects mentioned in this chapter and throughout the rest of this book. Cancer of the ovaries or cervix is still possible if just the uterus is removed, so awareness of this is very important.

HYSTERECTOMY ALTERNATIVES

Dr. Risa Kagan, a prominent, leading OB-GYN, as well as a menopause and fertility specialist in Berkeley, tells us: "More than 650,000 women undergo hysterectomies every year. Up to one-third of these surgeries are for abnormal menstrual bleeding which may be associated with hormone imbalances or growths in the uterine wall, such as fibroids or benign growth of endometrial tissue. Sometimes there is no apparent cause."

Statistics reveal that most women who have removal of the uterus are young, ending the chance of childbearing; three out of five of these surgeries involve women between the ages of fourteen and forty-four. It is argued that between 80 and 90 percent of these hysterectomies could be avoided by first trying more conservative measures, but other options often aren't discussed with women who are told that certain surgical procedures are necessary. On the other hand, there are serious medical reasons why hysterectomy, total hysterectomy, or oophorectomy can be the only life-saving decision.

Dr. Kagan continues: "Many women who are perimenopausal are looking for an alternative to hysterectomy. Low-dose oral contraceptive pills are now found to be safe and effective to control dysfunctional uterine bleeding for those who find them tolerable. Women can take them throughout the perimenopause as long as they are in generally good health and do not smoke.

"Outpatient surgical alternatives to hysterectomy are now available with operative hysteroscopy. [Hysteroscopy involves inserting a small, bright light and a thin telescope into the vagina to illuminate the uterine cavity, either for examination or surgery.] These options include burning the lining of the uterus, known as endometrial ablation, and the removal of fibroids, a process called myomata resection. These are safe, less invasive, and less expensive alternatives to hysterectomy. Research efforts are under way to further simplify these procedures which may enable them to be performed in the office setting. These are ideal procedures for a woman in her forties who has completed childbearing and is experiencing excessive bleeding as a symptom of her perimenopause."

Uterine balloon therapy and Outpatient Endometrial Resection and Ablation (OPERA) are two recent procedures that can be performed in an OB-GYN office to cure excessive uterine bleeding that compromises a woman's quality of life. Dr. Brian Walsh of Brigham and Women's Hospital in Boston says, "They are only for the woman who is not going to become pregnant, because they destroy the lining that would be necessary to nourish a pregnancy, and they would not be used to treat fibroids or cancer." These office treatments are more convenient than the ablation mentioned above and would not require going into a hospital surgical situation.

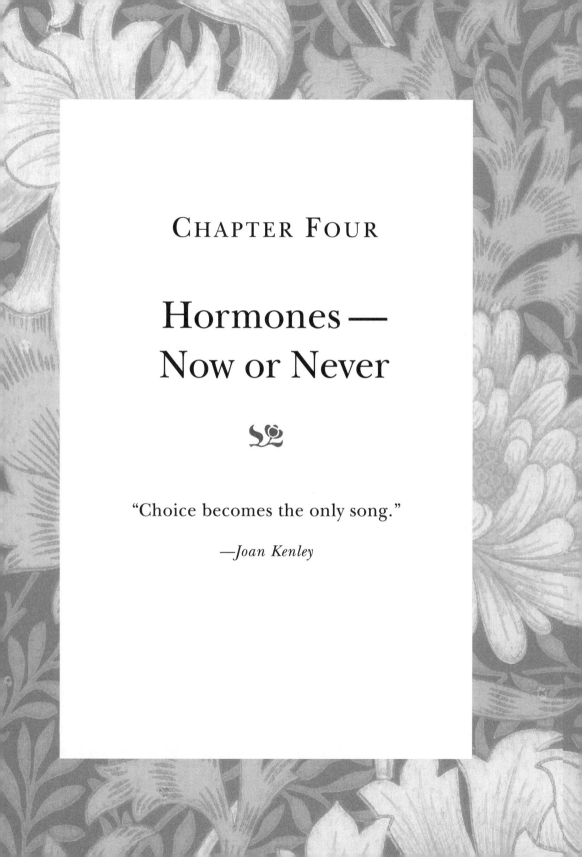

CHAPTER FOUR

Hormones — Now or Never

❧

"Choice becomes the only song."

—*Joan Kenley*

REPRODUCTIVE SYSTEM

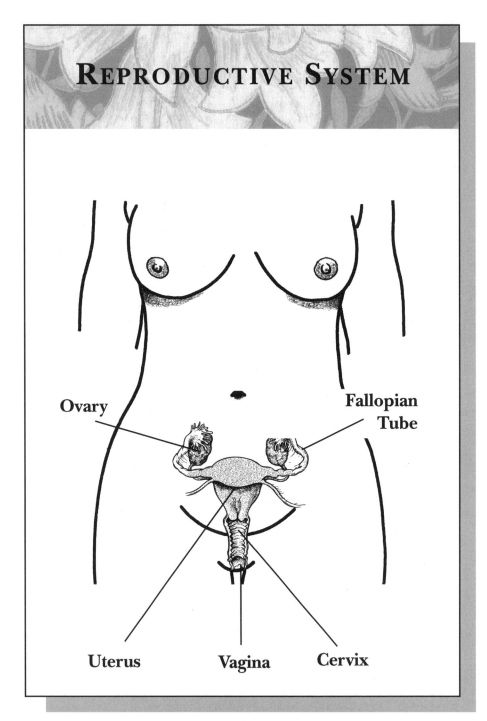

Ovary

Fallopian
Tube

Uterus   Vagina   Cervix

Source: American Cancer Society. Design by Roland Gauthier.

HORMONES — NOW OR NEVER

≈

*P*amela says, "I'd have no life at all without hormone therapy." Her older sister Kim agrees. Donna contends, "I wouldn't dream of tampering with the natural aging process by choosing to take hormones, no matter what anyone says!" Her mother died of estrogen-dependent breast cancer after taking large doses of estrogen-alone therapy prescribed in the sixties. Mary Ann confesses, "I'm so confused. There's no way I'll ever understand what to do." Her mother felt that talking about personal health matters was disgusting. Suzanne declares, "Nothing's bothering me, so I have nothing to worry about." Her Aunt Sara and her mom were healthy and lived long, vital lives, with no health problems.

These are just a few of the attitudes voiced by women every day. Unfortunately, most attitudes remain unchallenged. Opinions become beliefs. For the curious, health studies abound with conflicting information. What's published today can seem to oppose other findings released yesterday.

Who to trust? To treat or not to treat—for symptoms *or* prevention? What's safe to believe? These should be the burning questions before *any* opinions are rendered.

The most frequent statement I hear regarding hormones is, "I only want to take something *natural.*" But there's a great deal of confusion about what is "natural." There's only one answer. It's any substance that mirrors your own chemistry. If hormone products start out using wild yams, for instance, they still have to be compounded to match the estrogen, progesterone, or testosterone produced by your body. So even though this process happens in a laboratory, these hormone replacement products can still be considered natural. Without any activating ingredients, wild yam extracts by themselves simply have no therapeutic hormonal effect.

There are, of course, a tremendous number of preventive measures and treatment possibilities for after-thirty-five potential health risks, menopause symptoms, and over-fifty health problems.

You need to learn how to define your particular health picture so you can customize your action plan.

Studies report that many women receive treatment programs from their health practitioners, yet there are a surprising number who never fill their prescriptions or begin the regimens. This behavior can put women at risk for potentially serious health problems. It certainly avoids any relief for the symptoms or concerns that took them to their health provider in the first place.

Once you begin any treatments that don't involve regular appointments, set up a check-in schedule with your health advisor every three to six months to report how you're doing, even when the status is "just fine." Keeping this line of communication open can give you the opportunity to ask, "What's new? What could update my regimen?"

Know also that with any program, some small percentage of women need up to a year of fine-tuning. Over the first month or two, you'll want to notice any improvements. Also observe any adverse side effects. If there are any, ask your advisor to consider changing the strength of any supplements, medications, or even treatment directions. Insist that you be given sufficient time to discuss this process with the health advisor or the informed patient-advocate or nurse practitioner in the office where your treatment journey begins.

TAKING CHARGE OF TREATMENT OPTIONS

This time of your life isn't like being lost in the woods, where the right thing to do is sit still and wait for someone to come along and find you. Women get lost because they don't get moving. They get lost when they believe the first suggested treatment will solve all their symptoms and concerns. It might, but it's unlikely, simply because your body is always in a state of change. You want a health practitioner who takes this reality into consideration as well as your knowledge, feelings, questions, and fears. Important surveys show that many women aren't aware of the treatment options available to them, and they don't think they can change treatments once they start. The idea that all women should use the same treatment is like saying they should all wear the same size, style, and color of shoes.

Certainly this book will help you to alleviate some degree of confusion. Explore these subjects with professionals and friends. Read up-to-date articles. Take responsibility for your treatment. Visit a health practitioner or clinic specializing in midlife and menopause issues. Ask questions. Know your options. Choose one. Try it. If it doesn't work for you, talk to your health advisor and make plans to make an adjustment. If needed, change doctors or clinics. And it will help if you can make the change with certainty, ignoring any grief or guilt about trying — optimistically — another direction,

Some women start with hormone replacement therapy, try it for only a short time, and move on to something else. Some are long-term users. Some choose hormone-free therapies altogether. Some try both.

So don't just sit there in the dark. Use the know-how you're learning here to light your way. Enjoy your hike out of the woods!

NON-HORMONAL TREATMENT OPTIONS

Choice is what treatment should be about. Choice gives us power over our own bodies and lives. A recent Gallup survey found that 80 percent of medical doctors talked to their women patients in a very limited way about health concerns, prevention, or the advantages of hormone replacement therapy, and less than 2 percent talked to them about non-hormonal treatment options. If your health advisor doesn't offer the choices you want, find one who does. There are more and more menopause specialists today who make it their business to know all the options. They can help you.

Women who enjoy good health and have other positive genetic factors that put them at low risk for heart disease, cancer, and osteoporosis may find that the only "treatments" they need are appropriate eating habits, regular exercise, calcium supplements, moderation in caffeine, alcohol, sugar, and fat intake, and no cigarette smoking, combined with ongoing monitoring of bone density and other possible physical changes. Women not on hormone replacement therapy also must have their bones, heart, thyroid, and blood monitored on an ongoing basis to be health-wise.

Just aging alone can cause vaginal dryness. It just comes with the territory. Water-based products are best. Replens®, Vagasil Intimate Moisturizer®, KY Long-Lasting Vaginal Moisturizer®, and Gyne-Moisturin® are four such moisture-producing products with non-prescription ingredients. These vaginal inserts can be placed three to four times a week to improve vaginal conditions for health reasons and for more comfortable sexual intercourse. Vagasil Intimate Moisturizer® is a cream that can soothe redness and itching. Astroglide® is an excellent vaginal lubricant to use during sexual activity.

For hot flashes, remedies can include slow breathing; vaginal or oral Vitamin E or Vitamin A; soy, black cohosh, or red clover plant estrogen products; or wild yam extract creams, which, however, must contain micronized progesterone to activate any progesterone effects in the body.

For joint problems and certain arthritis symptoms, two over-the-counter supplements, glucosamine sulfate and chondroitin sulfate, in combination, have relieved pain and stopped certain degeneration.

A variety of other symptoms can be relieved using plant and herbal supplements with estrogen-like qualities. Ginseng root, don quai, damiana, chasteberry, licorice root, and black cohosh, for instance, are found in teas, tinctures, and/or capsules. Yams and soybean-rich diets that include tofu, miso, and soy milk belong to the phytoestrogen food category. These plant estrogen-containing foods may have a positive effect for your complaints, but they may be too weak to make a dramatic difference if your symptoms are severe. Experiment with the type and quantity of various foods to know what actually makes you feel better.

Anxiety, phobias, moodiness, and sleeplessness can be relieved or healed with certain herbs, supplements, and tinctures. Psychological therapy, bodywork disciplines, behavior modification, and massage treatments may also be considered. Melatonin and mild herbal tranquilizers, including valerian root, are over-the-counter remedies that can be helpful for jangled nerves or sleep disturbance.

Mood-enhancement medications like Prozac®, Zoloft®, Paxil®, Effexor®, Serzone®, and Wellbutin® can be helpful for certain emotional or behavioral problems when other solutions don't work. Prozac, Paxil, and Serzone appear to have a greater incidence of limiting sexual desire than first thought when introduced. Effexor and Wellbutin have the least sexual side effects. Prescription drugs for these concerns should be taken under the watchful eye of a licensed mental health practitioner.

A word of warning: Women with menopause symptoms are sometimes prescribed tranquilizers or mood-altering drugs because of the behavior stimulated by the drop in estrogen levels. Menopause may also be misdiagnosed as fibromyalgia, chronic fatigue syndrome (CFS), or Epstein Barr disease, because the symptoms can be very similar.

ACUPUNCTURE, HOMEOPATHY, NATUROPATHIC AND NUTRITIONAL THERAPIES

These treatment options are among the most common non-hormonal therapies women choose for menopausal symptoms such as hot flashes, sleep problems, headaches, emotional ups-and-downs, and low energy, as well as various diseases and chronic complaints. It is reported that following these regimens can help to keep a person more in balance and more resistant to illness.

These methodologies, as well as other alternative options, follow the philosophy of focusing on the whole person from a body, mind, inter-personal, and social context. These practices are directed toward treating the cause of the problem, not just the symptoms.

The regimens are aimed at prevention, treating chronic ailments, and achieving sustained wellness, whereas standard medicine is more often focused toward eliminating symptoms, managing acute illness, and performing surgeries. However, it is becoming more and more popular to treat patients with a combination of both standard and alternative methods.

The Chinese medical practice of **acupuncture** has been around for more than 2,500 years. The practitioners use seeing, hearing, smelling, and touching to focus on a patient's condition. Most importantly, they are skilled in the diagnostic observation of the tongue and sensitive evaluation of the wrist pulse, which they find can reveal a disease when it is just beginning, sometimes up to five years before any symptoms are detectable.

Homeopathy, which uses tiny oral doses of flower, herb, or other extracts to help stimulate the body's own healing process, was developed by a German doctor in the 1700s. The remedies are chosen based on a detailed personal and health history along with certain behavioral and emotional traits. Some of the treatment choices used for menopause are Lachesis®, Lycopodium®, Natrum Muriaticum®, Nux Vomica®, Pulsatilla®, and Sepia®. Homeopathic remedies are dispensed by homeopathic physicians and clinics, and they are also available in weaker doses at health food stores.

Naturopathic and **nutritional therapies** are used by those who want to address dietary deficiencies, weak immune systems, and the prevention of illness, in addition to employing "natural" methods for curing ailments. The intention is to plan treatments that do not cause negative reactions or risks to the patient. These therapies call on the healing energy that is viewed to be present in everyone, and they use the broad consideration of the mental, emotional, physical, and spiritual perspectives.

The alternative or complementary therapies mentioned above, as well as many others listed in "Alternative Treatment Options" at the end of this book, offer a wide range of choices. Unfortunately, only a tiny fraction of the money spent on standard medical research has been allotted to evaluate these healing approaches. Consequently, there haven't been clinical studies run to show whether and to what extent alternative treatments benefit the patient. More recently, interest has grown and some funding has become available to establish needed research. Today more and more medical doctors are beginning to see the curative potential of complementary treatments or combining of several approaches.

The best answer for you? To know about both medical and alternative options and to find a health care provider who will talk to you about the advantages and limitations of both. When choosing combination treatments, be sure they are designed in a way that will be truly complementary and cause no harm.

HORMONE REPLACEMENT THERAPIES

Estrogen, progesterone, and small amounts of the male sex hormone testosterone are all produced by the female ovaries. Hormone production decreases beginning in a woman's mid-to-late thirties to early fifties and can be "replaced" by hormone therapies.

The current definitions are as follows:
- ERT = Estrogen Replacement — estrogen alone.
- HRT = Estrogen/Progesterone Hormone Replacement Therapy — estrogen and progesterone in some combination.

Testosterone Replacement Therapy can be prescribed with either or both hormone replacement therapies or as a single hormone treatment by itself. The various ways you can take these hormones are detailed later in this chapter.

HORMONE REPLACEMENT DECISIONS

Hormone replacement therapy is the most debated topic in the field of menopause. Should you? Shouldn't you? How much? How long? Starting when? Most of the controversy is about estrogen. Research tells us that 85 percent of you will experience some menopausal symptoms such as hot flashes, vaginal dryness, sleeplessness, mood swings, short-term memory loss, etc., but most likely not all of them.

There are women with no symptoms who take hormones to prevent the serious risk of heart disease, bone fractures, and other major health problems that can occur after menopause.

Estrogen supplements can be very important for pre-menopausal women who have their ovaries surgically removed because this procedure creates an instant menopause.

Many women and a great number of health professionals call hormone replacement a "miracle cure" for everything from hot flashes to "the blahs," from change in sexual interest to breaking into tears at the market. Women choosing hormone therapy may take a combination of all three hormones or other appropriate mixes. Some women say HRT makes them feel worse, and no customizing succeeds. There are certain circumstances when women should not consider estrogen replacement, and these conditions are discussed later in the chapter.

For hot flashes, sleep disorders, and other symptoms, some women find that using progesterone alone helps. For others, testosterone may be the treatment choice for managing hot flashes, feeling energized, alert, and sexual. DHEA-sulfate, an abundant hormone secreted by the adrenal glands that declines with aging, appears, in supplementation therapy, to have some protective influences for certain diseases, joint pain, menopause symptoms, and the immune system. Interest in dhea hormone replacement is growing among doctors, researchers, and patients.

There are those who are against any treatment for menopause that's "medical," feeling there haven't been enough "official" long-term studies to have confidence in the safety of any hormone replacement regimen. On the other hand, there have been no official long-term trials on "alternative" treatments.

The reason hormones are replaced, whether or not you have symptoms, is because of the important effects they have on your health: bones, heart, blood vessels, skin, reproductive and urinary functions, the brain, endocrine system, mucous membranes, and more. Hormones also affect your moods and energy. During your midlife transition period, a significant reduction in estrogen, progesterone, and testosterone can upset your mind, body and spirit. This hormonal reduction can trigger other health problems as well. Think about how the information applies specifically to you. Make certain to select a health advisor you trust and would want to stay with over time. Take some time to mull it all over.

When you feel comfortable with your personal decision about whether hormone replacement or non-hormonal health management is for you, make the choice with confidence. Give that choice a fair trial. Give it time to have it adjusted to your individual needs before you reject it or become discouraged. Always know that any choice you make can be changed. Your search for more answers can and should go on.

Remember that new developments about what's known and what's treatable are emerging all the time.

DETAILED ESTROGEN INFORMATION

Estrogen can be defined as a group of body-regulating hormones (estradiol, estrone, and estriol) necessary for female sexual development and for healthy functioning of the reproductive system. The whole idea of taking some form of estrogen replacement is to give back to your body a hormone supply no longer produced by your ovaries. Although you may not be aware of it, estrogen has regulated hundreds of important functions for you since puberty. Therefore, the loss of estrogen production can cause your body to go through a form of withdrawal. The debate about estrogen and breast cancer will be covered briefly here and in more detail in Chapter Six.

John C. Arpels, M.D., tells us, "Estrogen acts to help prevent all forms of cardiovascular disease and osteoporosis, lower blood sugar levels, activate some of the protective cells of the immune system, improve cholesterol levels, regulate brain function and overcome disturbing menopausal symptoms."

After all, your ovaries have been supplying estrogen naturally for about forty years. Until this century, most women died around the time of their menopause. Now women may live to be a hundred years old. This could be considered "unnatural" because so many hormones are shutting down, putting women at risk for disease without conscious intervention through preventive measures.

Estrogen advocates ask if your car came with a fifty-year gasoline supply, and currently has no incompatibility with gasoline, would you refuse to refuel after the fifty-first year when you've discovered it can run for fifty more?

On the other hand, there are medical experts and some alternative treatment practitioners who have a more conservative view. They feel that no estrogen replacement is wise under any circumstances or that only very short-term therapies are appropriate.

SOY, RED CLOVER, BLACK COHOSH, AND OTHER PLANT-BASED/ PLANT-MODIFIED ESTROGENS

Plant-based estrogens, known as phytoestrogens, are estrogenic plant substances compounded for estrogen replacement. The new, non-prescription, red clover-based Promensil® tablet developed in Australia are very useful for those women who cannot or do not want to take other forms of ERT and want to manage hot flashes, mood swings, and sleeplessness. The herb black cohosh has been documented in clinical trials in Germany to alleviate menopausal symptoms, and research is also under way in the US to study soy and other estrogenic herbs. Recently, don quai alone was found to be no better than placebos for treating hot flashes, but in traditional Chinese medicine it is compounded with other substances that can prove effective. None of these products, especially when they are purchased over-the-counter, should be used without expert professional advice.

New research shows that the plant-modified estrogens, Estrace® (estriadol B17) and Estratab® (esterified estrogens), in a low daily dose of 0.3 milligrams, can prevent hot flashes, osteoporosis, and lower the blood fats associated with 25 percent of heart disease cases. That dose can also be considered for treatment of urinary/genital tissue dryness caused by estrogen depletion. However, this regimen may not be strong enough to favorably affect other problems. At this point in time, most women take an estrogen hormone therapy that is derived from the urine of pregnant horses, Premarin®, and the dose is usually more than twice that in the plant-modified regimen used in this recent two-year study at the University of California in San Francisco.

Further studies are needed to determine the long-term effects of such a small dose of these plant-modified estrogens, but it's encouraging to note that there are fewer difficulties with vaginal bleeding, headaches, and nausea. If you have a uterus, it reduces the risk of uterine cancer and requires less frequent regimens of progesterone to shed the lining with a bleeding period than is the case when estrogen is prescribed in higher doses.

Plant estrogens are basically non-steroidal, although enzymes can be added to modify them into a steroid product. The hope is that future formulations of the non-steroidal type will be effective over an even wider spectrum for those women who should not take steroid hormones of any kind.

SERM—Designer Estrogens

"SERM" stands for selective estrogen receptor modulators, a relatively recent group of drugs that function somewhat like estrogen in protecting bones from osteoporosis without stimulating breast tissue. They do not cause buildup of the lining of the uterus or cause estrogen-dependent breast cancer tumors to grow more rapidly. Evista®, the brand name for raloxifene, the SERM from Eli Lilly, is now available by prescription. Even though very few side effects have been reported in the study groups, hot flashes can occur with varying degrees of severity. For some women in their sixties and seventies, there is less incidence of breast tenderness sometimes caused by estrogen. There is a good result in producing bone hip strength with SERMs. However, the lower spine effect is only 50 percent of that achieved with standard doses of ERT, but equal to the low dose of .03 milligrams of estrogen replacement just mentioned.

There is a good result in bone hip strength with SERM, but the lower spine effect is only 50 percent of standard ERT.

Vaginal and Urinary Tract ERT

Estring®—a vaginal silicone ring—is a product that addresses vaginal and urinary/bladder health and should have made headlines when it finally became available recently in this country. For the first time, many women who can't take estrogen or who have been predisposed against replacement therapies that circulate estrogen in the body—or those who find their regular ERT dose needs a boost where these concerns are involved—can consider this convenient, no-mess product which delivers a consistent, low dose of estradiol to the urogenital area for up to three months per ring. In four to six weeks, the ring, inserted like a diaphragm, can increase vaginal lubrication and restore tissue resilience which in turn protects you from yeast infections and promotes more comfort sexually. Estring can also contribute to urinary tract health and reduce urinary urgency and bladder infections.

ESTROGEN THERAPY — REPORTED ADVANTAGES

It is recognized that women with moderate to severe menopausal symptoms or certain health risks such as heart disease, colon cancer, and osteoporosis should know the advantages of estrogen replacement as a treatment choice.

Not as widely reported are other advantages of estrogen therapy deemed valid by menopausal and health experts. Estrogen replacement is known and/or believed to:

- guard against heart disease and stroke, the major killers of women over fifty;
- decrease bone deterioration (osteoporosis);
- reduce hip fractures and spinal changes that cause dowager's hump and decreased height;
- raise heart-positive HDL cholesterol, improve blood flow, and prevent blood vessels from accumulating harmful plaque;
- enhance healthy functioning of internal organs, joints, and muscles;
- eliminate or reduce hot flashes, sleeping difficulties, night sweats, and the sensation of crawly, itchy skin;
- promote a sense of emotional well-being;
- improve midlife short-term memory loss;
- increase energy;

- keep skin more vital by increasing collagen and moisture content;
- prevent vaginal dryness plus thinning and shrinking of vaginal tissue;
- lower incidence of urinary tract infections and aid in bladder control;
- restore blood flow to sexual tissue, improving sexual response;
- prevent age-related mental conditions, such as the ability to retain and retrieve information, and offer protection against senile dementia and Alzheimer's; and
- protect eyes from cataracts and dryness.

Side effects of estrogen replacement can include nausea, breast tenderness, abnormal uterine bleeding, and headaches. These symptoms usually subside after one or two months. But if you have discomfort, it can indicate the prescription strength or type of estrogen is incompatible and adjustments are needed. There are women who do not feel comfortable with ERT, even after many attempts. In these cases, estriol — the weaker, less risk-prone estrogen — is an option for those who aren't candidates for the more standard ERT programs. Dr. Jonathan Wright's triestrogen formula combines estriol, estradiol, and estrone in an 80-10-10 percentage and is first prescribed at 2.5 mgs, then up to 5 mgs if required to relieve the symptoms. Phytoestrogen supplements can also be considered.

As Dr. Arpels tells us, "Menopausal medicine is concerned with maintaining optimal health and life quality as women mature. To the extent that many organ systems function best on some level of estrogen, replacing or supplementing this hormone has taken on the same philosophic and medical context as adding thyroid hormone or insulin when these are too low."

Ways to Take ERT

Estrogen is available in a variety of strengths and methods of delivery. Treatment should be customized for you, ordinarily beginning with the lowest dose indicated by your history and symptoms. You and your health advisor can decide from that initial dosage what your symptom responses suggest about tolerance, strength, or form. Estrogen is taken daily or, in some regimens, twenty-five out of thirty days. However, most experts feel that estrogen's benefits are more reliable if taken every day.

Estrogen is available in:

1) pills—swallowed; absorbed under the tongue; placed in vagina.

2) skin patches—adhesive patches that can deliver continuous, steady amounts of estradiol are usually worn on the lower abdomen, hip, or thigh area, but can be placed anywhere on the body that is convenient except the breasts. Climara patches can be cut to customize the dose, are easy on the skin, and only need changing weekly. Vivelle, a three-to-four day patch has a somewhat better adhesive with less lint collection around the edges. In some circumstances it can be reapplied if it comes off and can be cut to adapt the dose. FemPatch comes in one low dose of .025 mg and is changed weekly. Estraderm patches are changed every 3 to 4 days as well, but they can't be cut to adjust dosage and aren't as thin. The dose delivery is more uneven than the first two.

Hormone Replacement Medication

Trade Name	Generic Name	Source
Estrogens		
Premarin	Conjugated equine estrogens	Urine of pregnant mares
Estratab, Menest	Esterlied estrogens	Modified plant estrogens
Estrace	*Estradiol	Modified plant estrogens
Ogen, Ortho-est	Estrone estropipate	Modified plant estrogens
Promesil	Phyto-estrogen (phenolic)	Modified plant estrogens
Vivelle, Climara, Alora Fem-patch (adhesive skin patches)	*Estradiol	Modified plant estrogens
Progestogens		
Provera, Cycrin	Medroxyprogesterone acetate (MPA)	Synthesized from soy
Aygestin	Norethindrone acetate	Modified plant hormone
Prometrium	*Micronized progesterone	Modified plant hormone
Progest IUD (intrauterine device)	Time-released progesterone	Modified plant hormone
Crinone (vaginal cream)	Progesterone	Modified plant hormone
Combinations		
Prempro	Conjugated estrogens and MPA	Premarin and MPA in single pill
Premphase	Conjugated estrogens and MPA	Two pills: Premarin, followed by Premarin with MPA
Estratest	Esterified estrogens and methyl-testosterone	Modified Plant compound
Other		
Evista	Raloxifene	Selective estrogen receptor modulator

Starred items are products that mirror a woman's own hormone chemistry.

3) creams — applied topically for vaginal dryness and urinary problems; normally safe in very low doses for those not able to take estrogen otherwise.

4) gels — pre-measured doses from pump dispensers can be applied easily to skin and may be available soon in the U.S.; raise circulating blood levels more than skin patches, but twenty-four-hour delivery is not as sustained as the patches.

5) pellets — tiny implants (buttock or lower abdomen) injected into the fatty tissue under the skin which last three–four months; sometimes problem with removal if side effects occur; are mostly chosen when other estrogen methods can't be used.

6) vaginal silicone ring — a ninety-day vaginal insert sold as Estring, which does not increase the level of circulating estrogen and can keep or restore normalcy to dry vaginal tissue and prevent or cure some types of urinary incontinence.

Estrogen replacement taken under the tongue or placed in the vagina is three to four times more potent than the same dose swallowed in a pill. If you change to one of these methods, be careful to adjust the dose. It is easy to get dependent on higher doses of estrogen. Therefore, it's better to stabilize at the lowest dose possible, inasmuch as it can be difficult to cut back.

An example of customizing treatment is to see whether a woman needs to increase her estrogen dose slightly during the days she is taking progesterone. Progesterone acts as a suppressant for estrogen and possibly her requirements for estrogen may need to be adjusted accordingly. Symptoms will tell. Another concern that should not be ignored is for the woman who experiences uncomfortable withdrawal symptoms when using the older regimen of going "off" estrogen for five days each month. She should be updated to continuous estrogen.

Drug companies make various estrogen compounds. For instance, Estrace® is a brand name for estradiol, an estrogen that mirrors your own body's estrogen makeup. Its source is wild yams. More widely prescribed is Premarin®, the estrogen product made from horse (equine) estrogens. It has been available for many years and is derived from pregnant mares' urine. Ogen® is the brand name for estrone replacement, which is also derived from yams.

Right now, doctors usually prescribe estrogen alone only for those women who have had surgical removal of the uterus, or uterus and ovaries, barring other health risks covered in the next few pages. Otherwise, estrogen is combined with progesterone as detailed later on in the chapter. When you take estrogen in pill form, take it at the same time each day. If taken with food, it will be absorbed better.

Have your health advisor consider contacting any of the reputable Alternative Pharmacies mentioned in the back of this book for further ways to approach estrogen or other hormonal replacement.

The choice of which estrogen compounds and delivery methods are right for you should be made after you consider the options mentioned in this chapter.

REASONS NOT TO
TAKE ESTROGEN THERAPY

No medication or treatment is risk-free for everyone—medically, emotionally, or physically. A small percentage of women have few, if any, menopause symptoms and no health risks that might indicate hormonal replacement. Some women taking hormones have side effects that can't be managed. Some just don't want medical meddling in what they see as a natural process. Others don't choose estrogen replacement because they don't know enough about the pros and cons, or because their practitioner hasn't taken the time educate them about the possible health benefits. Women also have fears about hormone replacement because of the negative publicity created by:

1) the high doses of estrogen given to women in the past;

2) the false equation with birth control pills that can be many, many times stronger; and,

3) the sometimes inaccurate information that proliferates in the media.

Women should not take estrogen if they presently have breast or uterine cancer, certain ovarian cancers, recent heart attack, current or past melanoma skin cancer, or unexplained vaginal bleeding.

Women who may be able to take estrogen with careful consideration are those who have uterine fibroids, phlebitis, liver or gall bladder disease, and trouble with blood clotting. It's important to seek expert medical advice because estrogen replacement may or may not have an adverse effect on these pre-existing conditions. It depends on the woman's history, the new information about estrogen's effect on these disorders, and what form of estrogen is used — all very important considerations.

In the past, the preceding list included diabetes, but Dr. Arpels tells us that "Estrogen actually improves insulin availability and glucose transport."

Those who smoke need to realize that smoking and estrogen are not a good mix. Smoking suppresses some of the positive effects of ovarian-produced estrogen or estrogen replacement by neutralizing its usefulness in the body.

Of course, smoking greatly increases the risk of lung cancer. Lung cancer is second only to heart disease in causing death for women over fifty. Smokers also put themselves at great risk for heart disease, osteoporosis, and many other serious health problems.

No matter what the potential risks, women suffering from severe menopausal symptoms, and who get no relief from non-hormonal treatments, may choose short-term estrogen therapy. It can help to keep some measure of positive quality of life for them until the peak symptom phase of their transition is over—an average time of three to five years.

If the decision is made to stop estrogen replacement after an extended period of use, the estrogen dose should be lowered very slowly—over two to three months—in order to minimize withdrawal reactions. Once estrogen is discontinued, some symptoms will most likely return. The medical benefits for disease prevention will cease.

ESTROGEN REPLACEMENT CONTROVERSIES

Estrogen has had an up-and-down history. It was hailed as a wonder cure during the sixties and seventies. The message was, "Take it! Be a young woman forever!" At that time, doctors prescribed estrogen replacement alone and in much higher doses than currently recommended. It is not part of the estrogen and progesterone programs appropriate for most women today. In the past, with high doses of estrogen alone, some women developed cancer of the uterine lining. Evidence pointed to a connection between the high doses of estrogen and the cancer. Estrogen got a bad reputation. This pattern is similar to the early history of high-dose birth control pills, which also initially used a very potent form of estrogen and were connected to certain medical risks.

Today, estrogen is used in much lower doses. And for women who still have their uterus intact, ERT needs to include taking a form of progesterone in a suitable manner to reduce the risk of endometrial cancer. The "Progesterone and ERT" section in this chapter discusses the ways progesterone/progestin can be combined with estrogen.

Research indicates that women who take hormone replacement therapy have a lower risk for ovarian and endometrial cancer than women who don't. Many medical experts now are making arguments in favor of estrogen replacement for women whose medical profiles indicate a need for it because of its disease prevention benefits and quality of life enhancement. Even so, no one should choose a treatment without feeling it's appropriate.

ERT AND BREAST CANCER

There is indeed a great debate about breast cancer and estrogen replacement. There is no research that proves taking estrogen is directly responsible for causing breast cancer. It is true that if you already have a cancerous breast tumor, estrogen-dependent or estrogen non-dependent, estrogen replacement can make that tumor grow faster. Many experts say that women with any kind of breast cancer should not consider estrogen supplements. Women who have a family history of two first-degree relatives — mother or sisters — with breast cancer should talk seriously with their health advisors before choosing hormone replacement.

In her book *Understanding Breast Cancer,* Patricia Kelly, Ph.D., medical geneticist and at John Muir Medical Center in Northern California, points out that according to one of the eight studies on the subject: "Among women diagnosed with breast cancer at age fifty or older, those who were taking replacement estrogens prior to their diagnosis had a significantly improved survival rate compared to non-users. A contributing factor could be that women taking estrogen are under closer medical supervision."

In addition, the studies Kelly examined "generally find little . . . increase in risk of breast cancer with years of use [of replacement estrogens], even in women who have a family history of breast cancer." However, there are other studies that claim there is a slight increase of breast cancer in later years with long-term use. (See Chapter Six for more information on this important subject.)

ERT AND CHOLESTEROL

Estrogen has been shown to help many women in midlife control blood cholesterol levels, which tend to rise as estrogen levels fall during menopause. If you want to lower your cholesterol levels with estrogen replacement in the shortest amount of time, some of your regimen needs to be taken orally so that it can be processed through your liver. Conjugated equine estrogens like Premarin® can initially have faster results in lowering total cholesterol levels. However, other types of estrogen replacement with sufficient dosage can become equal in this effect after a year of use.

Dr. Arpels adds to our understanding: "Estrogen has a strong influence on the liver cells which manufacture cholesterol, raising the protective HDL, the 'good' cholesterol, and lowering the 'bad' LDL cholesterol. Estrogen replacement has an equally important role as a very powerful anti-oxidant, inasmuch as it keeps the LDL from turning 'bad' via oxidation."

ERT AND UTERINE CANCER

From the 1940s through the 1960s, estrogen replacement by itself — meaning without progesterone (or progestin) therapy — was connected to an increased risk of cancer of the uterus. Since the late 1960s, however, women who have a uterus have been advised not to take ERT alone, but in a prescribed regimen that provides some combination with progesterone.

When progesterone/progestin is prescribed for twelve to fourteen days each month along with estrogen, these two hormones mimic what the body does naturally before menopause: During this hormone-regulated cycle, the uterine lining builds up with the use of the estrogen replacement, then sloughs off with the progesterone regimen, mimicking menstruation. There is no increased risk of uterine cancer for women taking this form of HRT or the "continuous-combined" method which involves daily doses of both estrogen and progesterone. With this continuous-combined regimen there are no periods, although 40 to 60 percent of the women on it experience some irregular bleeding or spotting during the first six to twelve months of treatment. It is reported in at least four studies that estrogen with progesterone—using either regimen—actually lowers the risk of uterine cancer as compared with women not on HRT.

PROGESTERONE DEFINED

Progesterone is a sex hormone essential for healthy functioning of the female reproductive system. Before menopause, it is produced in the ovaries during the second half of the menstrual cycle to slough off the lining of the uterus and produce a period. This process keeps the uterine wall healthy. Small amounts of progesterone are also produced in the adrenal glands. Progesterone produces changes in the cervix and vagina during the menstrual cycle. It can affect moods and energy, producing the PMS symptoms some women have before their monthly periods — bloating and lack of energy as well as feelings that are "blue" and "blah."

Certain advocates of progesterone claim it can be used in hormone replacement therapy to protect bones from osteoporosis. This is not true. Calcium supplements can have more beneficial impact on bones than progesterone regimens.

PROGESTERONE CHOICES

Progesterone replacement is available in various types and methods of delivery. When manufactured from plant sources that mirror your own body's chemical make-up of this hormone, it is called natural, micronized progesterone. It has only been available for HRT in the last few years and is not usually available in drugstores. It can be prescribed by your physician and ordered from any of the Alternative Pharmacies listed in the back. Provera® is the brand name of the most well-known synthetic progesterone replacement. It is plant-derived, but chemically different from natural progesterone. Generically, this is called progestin or progestogen.

The products you can consider in each category are
Progesterone (natural):
　1) pills taken by mouth or under the tongue
　2) vaginal or rectal suppositories or tablets
　3) injection
Progestin/Progestogen (plant-modified):
　1) pills
　2) patch (presently under development in Europe)

Choosing injections of progesterone for hormone replacement is the least convenient method and can cause muscle soreness at the injection site for a percentage of women. However, for the management of heavy bleeding, it is often the preferred choice.

For those patients who cannot take estrogen and who want to eliminate hot flashes, two progestogens can be considered: Provera® and Megace®. The potency of Megace is four times the strength of Provera and is used as a treatment for estrogen-dependent breast cancer because it suppresses breast estrogen. In some circumstances, Megace can deplete estrogen in the body to the point that the estrogen receptors die.

There is concern that any progestin (e.g. Norethindrone®) dosage that is too strong for women with heart or blood vessel problems may be potentially harmful. It is possible that progestin can constrict blood vessels to the degree that a decrease in blood flow to the heart can occur and possibly cause a heart attack or stroke. If an episode of this kind takes place, an Estrace® (estradiol) tablet under the tongue should be taken immediately and repeated at necessary intervals. Both doctor and patient should know about this possibility.

PROGESTERONE AND ERT

Progesterone/progestin replacement, in some combination with estrogen (HRT), is most frequently prescribed as a cyclic monthly regimen by medical doctors to activate post-menopausal "menstruation" that sheds the uterine lining and prevents cancer of the uterus. Women who have had their uterus surgically removed don't need progesterone for this purpose, but might choose it for managing hot flashes if they aren't taking estrogen.

There are, however, ways to take progesterone without having monthly "periods." Originally, it was thought that this combination was necessary on a monthly basis. Now it is considered safe every two to three months, or for some, every six months. This way of looking at it has helped women who do not want to have regular thirty-day periods to consider hormone replacement more favorably. The progesterone replacement gets rid of the endometrial cancer risk by letting the body shed the uterine lining, much like pre-menopausal periods.

Progesterone/progestin can be combined with estrogen in these formats: for twelve days each month, for fourteen days every three to six months, or daily.

A daily estrogen/progesterone regimen is called "continuous-combined therapy." Some women find it attractive because there are no periods — the uterine lining doesn't build up with this regimen. Research has found this combination is not the best choice for every woman in the first three years of menopause because it has a 40 to 60 percent chance of causing break-through bleeding at unexpected intervals. Those who begin this at the fourth year may still have three to six months of irregular spotting before this therapy becomes effective. Since progesterone/progestin is given daily, this method may require more fine-tuning and in some cases, unpleasant symptoms can increase during the adaptation time. Many women, however, find it perfect.

Your individual choice should be determined by several considerations. First, you want to find the dosage and type of progesterone/progestin that is friendliest to your body and moods. The wrong compound or the wrong amount can make a difference. If a particular program isn't working, you can develop sore breasts, the blues, lack of energy, and bloating. For some women, switching from the stronger, synthetic progestin to the more natural, micronized form — one that chemically mirrors your body's progesterone — eliminates many side effects. Changing the dosage or switching to sublingual, vaginal, or rectal methods can help, too. You will find that the synthetic progestins are found in 2.5, 5, or 10 mgs, and the micronized form of progesterone supplements are prescribed in 100, 200, or 300 mgs. The reason for this is that the form which chemically mirrors your body's hormone takes a higher dosage to do the same work.

TESTOSTERONE REPLACEMENT

Testosterone is known as the male sex hormone. It's the hormone that makes a man a man, just as estrogen makes a woman a woman. It gives men body hair, sex drive, deep voices, and certain tendencies toward aggressiveness. Women produce a certain amount of testosterone, but not as much as men. During the reproductive years, this "male hormone" is produced in sufficient amounts by the ovaries and adrenal glands to give women a sex drive, muscle strength, and a certain sense of mental and physical "oomph."

When women enter menopause, most hormones, not just estrogen, take a dip. If your testosterone drops too low, the result can be loss of sexual interest, assertiveness, and/or energy, which can then cause difficulties in relationships at home and work. To counteract these symptoms, most women today who choose testosterone replacement take 1.25 mgs or less orally. It must be prescribed by a medical doctor. Testosterone also helps treat breast tenderness that sometimes accompanies hormone replacement therapy. There are women who choose a medically prescribed testosterone cream which is applied topically to the skin surrounding the vaginal opening — and to the clitoris, whether or not there is any shrink-age — to enhance sexual arousal.

There are three types of testosterone, all of which are based on soy sources and prepared in various ways to prevent enzymes from degrading or destroying the hormone as it enters your system:

1) methyl-testosterone
2) fluorinated testosterone
3) micronized testosterone

As with all medicines — including estrogen and progesterone — testosterone should be monitored. Normally, only very small doses are given to menopausal women to achieve positive results. If your physician is not versed in testosterone replacement, see that she/he is willing to learn about it. Prescribing blindly can result in uncomfortable side effects. If doses are too high, women may experience increased facial or body hair, thinning hair on the scalp, acne, weight gain, shrinking of the breasts — all reversible when the hormone replacement is stopped, except for non-reversible deepening of the voice. If a regimen is right, these symptoms do not occur. It's especially important to keep in regular contact with your health advisor about the benefits or drawbacks you notice when taking testosterone to discover whether the type or dosage is the one that is most reaction-free for you.

Steps for Receiving HRT

Before you start hormone treatment of any kind, your internist or gynecologist needs to take your medical history, perform a physical exam, and order a blood analysis and any other tests that may be indicated. Your hormone levels can be analyzed to indicate whether you may be entering or are in menopause. However, when it comes to hormone evaluation, your symptoms can often tell more than laboratory results. The "receptor sites" where hormones work may or may not be receiving and using the hormones your body is generating. Therefore, treatment should primarily be based on your personal experiences.

If you have your estrogen, progesterone, and testosterone levels checked, the blood test can also include what is known as your FSH (follicle-stimulating hormone) level. This is the pituitary sex hormone that signals your ovaries to release an egg each month. Since it's more and more difficult to get your egg follicles to react as menopause draws near, the pituitary gland will "try harder," pushing your FSH level upward.

It's important to remember that you may be having menopause-like symptoms and discomfort before your FSH level registers the so-called magic twenty-to-forty level used by physicians to indicate whether you are menopausal. Pre-menopausal women have levels that average between 5 and 20 mIU (milli-International Units).

CHOICES BEFORE BEGINNING HRT

Once you have chosen to begin a hormone program, your physician should customize a hormone replacement therapy for you which includes:
- type (source of hormone, i.e. yams, soy, mares' urine)
- dosage (strength of prescription)
- method of delivery (pills, patches, etc.)

• selection of hormones (estrogen, progesterone, testosterone)

Your treatment instructions—if you're not using the patch, which delivers a constant flow of replacement hormones—should include recommendations on the time of day you need it most based on your daily routines, symptoms, and sleeping patterns. Your medical advisor should monitor your regimen and how it is affecting you on a regular basis so your treatment can continue to be appropriate for your needs. Dr. Arpels, who is known for his expertise in fine-tuning hormone treatments, recommends: "Begin with the lowest doses to minimize initial start-up symptoms. For example, starting estrogen doses could be 0.25 mg for oral estradiol, 0.3 mg for conjugated equine estrogen, and 0.25 mg for the transdermal estradiol patch. For micronized progesterone, 300 mgs (100 mgs at breakfast and 200 mgs at bedtime), 5 mgs for progestin, and 0.625 mgs for testosterone, if needed."

The regimen can be adjusted every three to six weeks to reach the desired individual effect. If you have severe adverse reactions, which can include headaches, bloating, jitteriness, and depression, adjustments can be made as soon as these occur.

Sometimes estrogen and progesterone can actually work against each other. Some women experience an internal tug-of-war when the dosages are wrong. Well-known author Gail Sheehy, in her book *The Silent Passage*, writes, "Taking synthetic [progesterone] with the estrogen . . . was like pushing down the gas pedal and putting on the brakes at the same time, and it had left my body confused and worn out."

Always keep in mind that in addition to helping current symptoms or preventing future illness, you want to feel truly comfortable with your regimen, physically and emotionally.

If you take a prescription home and decide not to fill it, tell your doctor. If you don't like the way your initial hormone program makes you feel, find out what other possibilities might be better. It's a good idea to have a backup plan in mind with your physician when you begin your treatment so that you feel there's a safety net in place if you strike out on your first trial.

Also, be aware that your body may need a certain period of adjustment to any regimen you try. In most cases, when you and your physician have chosen a hormone replacement game plan, chances are you will feel just fine, although in some cases it can involve making small adjustments over the first three to five years, as the role played by the ovaries slowly diminishes. If you have made the decision to go the hormone route, stay with the program long enough to see what can work. Be patient. Don't stop cold turkey if you're not feeling well—it may shock your system. Find out from your health care provider a safe and comfortable way to gradually withdraw from your current regimen before you stop treatment altogether or begin another.

DURATION OF HORMONE REPLACEMENT THERAPY

In the past, when it has been prescribed mostly for relief from menopausal symptoms, two to five years of HRT was the norm, but opinions have changed. When experts consider the preventive benefits estrogen provides for osteoporosis, heart disease, cancer, and brain function, many recommend a fifteen-year to life-long regimen as more appropriate. Research for trials exceeding 26.8 years shows an overall significant decrease in health problems and premature deaths. The newest data says that even women seventy years old and beyond benefit from decreased cardiovascular risk when using ERT for an average of eighteen years.

PMS AND PRE-MENOPAUSAL SYMPTOMS

Hormone supplements and several non-hormonal treatment options can be prescribed for women who have the hardship of premenstrual syndrome (PMS) or who aren't yet in menopause, but who have menopause-like symptoms. There are choices to consider that require professional guidance.

Pre-menopausal women with symptoms may first seek non-hormonal therapies such as diet, exercise, stress reduction techniques, certain teas, nutritional supplements, primrose oil, vitamins, acupuncture, and other resources. This strategy is most common when the discomfort is not extreme.

Yet some women encounter their most severe menopausal difficulties long before they ever reach menopause. They might choose, under the care of their medical doctor, a low dose of estrogen taken by pill, patch, or vaginal application when unmanageable symptoms occur. This is sometimes called "estrogen supplementation" because this intermittent treatment is doing just that—enhancing what your body is still trying to do naturally, but can't with slowly-aging ovaries.

In certain cases, low-dose birth control pills (synthetic hormones) with a combination of estrogen and progestin or natural hormone compounds prescribed through Alternative Pharmacies can be used until you are menopausal. Hormone replacement therapy then becomes the better option because at this juncture, your own declining hormones are enhanced by HRT rather than being manipulated by the pill.

DHEA REPLACEMENT

DHEA is an abundant hormone secreted by the adrenal glands and ovaries. The production peaks in our late twenties and declines with age. According to some reports, it appears to provide protection against certain diseases, joint pain, memory loss, mood imbalances, low energy or libido, menopause symptoms, and attacks against the immune system. But wait before you dash out to take it! Have a careful respect for this treatment option if you decide to try it. Understand that the use of DHEA supplements should only follow research and conversations with your health advisor about the known pros and cons. DHEA is getting so much press and hype that even those who recommend it are cautious about the results to expect.

Women need to start any DHEA program with the very lowest dose — about 5 to 10 mgs — and build slowly up to 25 or 50 mgs by observing the reactions over a period of time. Too much DHEA can cause acne, breast soreness or swelling, and emotional reactions such as irritability or anger.

Micronized DHEA does not produce the same conversion to testosterone as the crystalline form, so it may be more easily tolerated and offer the desired effects with better reliability. Some feel that taking it under the tongue or vaginally produces better results than having it pass through the digestive system.

Over-the-counter DHEA may not have the potency you expect or the active ingredients you need unless you know the reliability of the brand you're buying; the information on the label can claim almost anything because there are no specific controls for these products. Your health counselor may provide you with the names of reputable brands, or order the DHEA for you through the one of the reputable Alternative Pharmacies we list in the back of the book or some other impeccable source.

≥℞

Hopefully, you now have some paths to lead you out of the woods of hormonal confusion. In recent years, significant and changing information has emerged every few months. Now it seems as if we are hearing about new ideas, theories, and products almost every week. Advice: Keep your eyes and ears alert.

CHAPTER FIVE

Hot Flashes
and Beyond

"Have you ever heard the sound

of one author shouting:

Prevent the problem.

Handle the problem.

Solve the problem?"

—*Joan Kenley*

Hot Flashes

*H*ot flashes are the most commonly known symptom of menopause — bothersome and legendary. Some women have them every hour, some once a month. You can have them only at night, only by day, or around the clock. They can be nothing more than "warm waves." Or they can be raging internal infernos that make you feel as if you'd like to dive into a pool of ice cubes. The flashes can last for seconds or minutes. They can happen anywhere, anytime — in bed, at the drugstore, at the office in the middle of a big business meeting. It's a time when "cool" takes on a whole new meaning.

Hot Flash Explained

Dr. Fredi Kronenberg is a physiologist specializing in women's health — menopause and hot flashes in particular — and Director of the Center for Complementary and Alternative Medicine at Columbia University. She explains that ". . . for some women, the hot flash means nothing more than an occasional, transient sensation of warmth; others, however, experience hourly waves of heat, drenching sweats, and increased heart rates. Hot flashes typically last three to six minutes, although they can be even shorter or last for more than thirty minutes."

Women may also experience chills and goose bumps after sweating, and it's not uncommon for some to have a sudden increase in heart rate, often sensed as palpitations. None of these sensations should be cause for alarm.

CAUSES OF HOT FLASHES

Apparently, hot flashes result from the actual withdrawal of estrogen rather than just from low estrogen levels. Some experts trace the origin of hot flashes to the hypothalamus which acts as a liaison between the brain and the rest of the body. These experts theorize that the hypothalamus may be involved in hot flashes and other vasomotor (blood vessel control) symptoms.

When you're having monthly periods, the rise in progesterone during the second half of the menstrual cycle raises the set-point of your hypothalamus which then raises your body temperature, making you feel warmer. Similarly, when you take progestogen, progestin, or a natural progesterone supplement, hot flashes may feel less severe because your body's thermostat is adjusted to a higher setting.

Many researchers believe that there are several triggers for hot flashes including stress or emotional turmoil, external heat sources, confining spaces, caffeine, and alcohol. It is also possible that certain foods such as sugar, hydrogenated or saturated fats, spicy or acidic foods, hot beverages, and large meals may trigger hot flashes for you.

WHO GETS HOT FLASHES

It is estimated that between 75 percent and 85 percent of American women experience hot flashes during menopause. However, according to Dr. Kronenberg, only

10 to 15 percent of women have frequent hot flash occurrences. The majority of women have only occasional flashes. She also notes that women with lower circulating estrogen levels often get hot flashes. However, low blood estrogen readings must be interpreted along with the consideration of your symptoms and how efficiently your estrogen receptors are processing the available estrogen.

Interestingly, a 1986 study by Y. Beyene reported that Japanese women rarely experience hot flashes and that Mayan women in Yucatan, Mexico, "do not report any symptoms at menopause other than menstrual cycle irregularity."

"HOT FLASH" AND "HOT FLUSH" DEFINED

The terms "hot flash" and "hot flush," as well as "night sweats," "power surges," and "warm waves" all basically refer to the same phenomenon. Most women describe a hot flash as the onset of a warm to hot feeling in the face, neck, and chest, which sometimes causes mild to severe sweating. A hot flush can refer to the rosy color that occurs on the face, neck, and chest. To be a little more explicit, a hot flash doesn't cause blushing of the skin or noticeable sweating — it's what you experience personally. A flush is what others notice when you begin to blush or glow.

SWEATING, NERVOUSNESS, AND IRRITABILITY

Heavy night sweats are really rough. If you can't keep your bedroom cool enough to reduce the intensity of your episodes — and if you aren't trying any treatments — you may want to take a cool shower or wrap soft cool-packs around your wrists and ankles before you retire. Wear cotton nightgowns or pajamas—or nothing. You can consider micronized progesterone pills, creams, or suppositories. Provera® and Megace® are synthetic progesterone choices. Or, if you prefer, try estrogen replacement therapy.

Up to 80 percent of menopausal women report—with varying degrees of intensity—that they feel nervous and irritable. Add to that repeated awakenings and loss of refreshing sleep and you have the perfect recipe for cranky or emotional reactions. As mentioned earlier, the changes in your hormones also affect your mood of the moment. Lifestyle adjustments and avoiding the food triggers mentioned in this chapter, plus hormonal or non-hormonal therapies, can improve or eliminate your problems.

DURATION OF HOT FLASHES

If you're afraid that these uncomfortable flashes will just never stop, don't worry—they probably won't last for the rest of your life. The prevalence of hot flashes is highest in the first two years of menopause, and then there usually is a decrease over time. Most women experience hot flashes for six months to two years, but some women have hot flashes which can continue for ten, twenty, or even forty years. Fortunately, fewer than 25 percent of women suffer with them beyond five years and only 10 percent have hot flashes for ten years or more.

Inasmuch as there are more women speaking openly about their hot flashes than ever before, there is a much greater chance that relief will be sought from medication, hormone replacement, alternative remedies, and/or behavioral modification.

HORMONE REPLACEMENT AND HOT FLASHES

Although estrogen has been used more frequently to control hot flashes, progesterone can also work for some women. Although the exact dynamic of estrogen replacement isn't scientifically determined, it is believed to influence the body's temperature-regulating system by somehow reducing the number and/or intensity of hot flashes. Normally it eliminates them altogether. Available for the first time in May 1998 is a breakthrough, over-the-counter plant estrogen tablet by Novogen called Promensil®, which is highly effective in controlling hot flashes with no known side effects.

Keep in mind that hormone replacement therapy may take two weeks before you start feeling relief from your hot flashes. The maximum effect may take as many as four weeks. At that point, if you don't get the results you want, you should speak with your physician about changing the dosage or type of therapy.

NATURAL METHODS TO CONTROL HOT FLASHES

There are some options for relieving and reducing your hot flashes by natural methods in addition to the natural plant estrogen just mentioned. Some may work better than others. Decide by a process of experimentation which remedies are most helpful since what helps one woman may not help another. Consider acupuncture, homeopathic and naturopathic treatments, vitamin therapy, a daily diet rich in soy products, and any other aids your health advisor may propose. You might also try the following suggestions:

- Carry a pocket fan.
- Learn what triggers your hot flashes by keeping a diary. Consider the time(s) of day you have the most distress. Then experiment with the kind of changes that will offer relief in these situations.
- If emotionally charged or stressful situations seem to encourage your hot flashes, pursue techniques to reduce the intensity of your emotional reactions. Slow down your breathing and learn some deep-breathing methods. Regular exercise can also reduce hot flashes for some individuals.
- Keep your work and home environments at a temperature cool enough to notice a difference, particularly when napping or sleeping. It is suggested that 65°F is effective in many cases. Often the more intense hot flashes or feelings of being too warm occur at night; results may be interrupted sleep as well as sleep deprivation difficulties, loss of concentration, moodiness, depression, etc.

HOT FLASHES AND AURAS

Studies have shown that immediately prior to the onset of a hot flash—within five to sixty seconds before—many women experience a premonition or "aura" of an impending episode. It's during this time that a subtle increase in heart rate and blood flow to the skin—particularly the hands and fingers—can occur. This may increase your consciousness that your body is about to have its "hot happening" even before noticeable symptoms appear. Use this premonition to your advantage with the techniques mentioned in this chapter to curb the intensity of your hot flashes.

NATURAL REMEDIES FOR HOT FLASHES

A number of natural teas and botanical and herbal substances have proved to be very effective hot flash treatments for some women and not for others. There is a long list of suggestions in the charts in the back of the book, including don quai, ginseng, damiana, Vitamin E, and natural progesterone creams. Most of these remedies have not been studied rigorously due to lack of funding, and it is important to remember that natural substances can be toxic if taken in excess. Always consult someone who is knowledgeable in these products to guide you to safe choices, always including how much and how often in the recommendation. Then experiment to see what specific remedies help your "Power Surges!"

INCONTINENCE

Incontinence difficulties can erode your confidence and chip away at your self-esteem. How can you be yourself if you're constantly worried about the possibility of an embarrassing accident? You may even feel you can't talk to your doctor about this "indelicate" subject. So you literally grin and bear it and put your life on hold. Don't.

URGENCY TO URINATE

If you feel a frequent urgency to urinate, and maybe leak when you laugh or sneeze, you are not alone. This is an important concern to address. The urinary frequency and incontinence symptoms that you are having are also bothering more than ten million other Americans — mostly women — to a greater or lesser degree.

Urinary problems can strike women at any age because of the effects of childbearing or the position of the uterus. Other considerations are the way women are built inside, diseases, infections, or weakness in the bladder and urinary tract. Many times the difficulty is caused by a decrease in estrogen.

Here are several types of urinary incontinence affecting bladder control:

1) Urge incontinence. The loss of bladder control stemming from various causes. Conditioned responses and bladder spasms can be triggered by various situations. An ordinary trigger, for instance, is the sound of running water. Urge incontinence can also be caused by infection of the urinary tract, estrogen decline during menopause, bladder inflammation, injuries to the spinal cord, pelvic irritation, spinal nerve-root problems, and chemotherapy. It is characterized by a powerfully urgent need to urinate, with loss of urine when one cannot reach the bathroom in time.

2) Stress incontinence. The leaking of urine when coughing, laughing, sneezing, or lifting puts pressure on the bladder. This stress response in the bladder can be affected by some of the conditions mentioned above. This is the most common urinary problem reported.

3) Overflow incontinence. Urine leaks out when the bladder is too full, though with no perceived sensation to urinate. This is often due to diabetes or spinal cord nerve injury.

Sad to say, a great number of women continue to have these difficulties because they are embarrassed or ashamed to get help. And help is available. I hope more women will be willing to talk about incontinence as millions of baby-boomer women sweep into midlife together. Whether you leak urine when you laugh, cough, or sneeze, have to go to the bathroom every hour, or ever lose control, be aware that:

- your estrogen levels may be low;
- the amount of collagen in your tissues could be decreasing;
- your bladder might have shrunk;
- your bladder may be having spasms;
- your pelvic floor muscles have become weaker;
- you could have a vaginal or urinary tract infection;
- you may have bladder cancer (although this is rare);
- certain commonly used medications can cause bladder problems, i.e., antihistamines, tranquilizers, and blood pressure medications; and
- spicy foods and caffeine beverages can affect bladder control.

REMEDIES FOR INCONTINENCE

Any or all of your incontinence difficulties, if not caused by major illness; injury; or structural conditions, can be solved or greatly improved with certain estrogen treatments, exercises, or behavior modification. (As a last recourse, choose antispasmodic drugs or surgery.)

Estrogen replacement therapy, topical estrogen at the urinary opening, or vaginal estrogen inserts such as tablets, suppositories, or the ninety-day vaginal ring sold under the brand name Estring®.

Biofeedback training clearly helps to retain certain muscles for effective urinary control. To attain the most efficient results, incontinence clinics and some urologists' offices offer this technology along with Kegel exercises, detailed next.

Kegel exercises. A recent study supports the premise that strengthening the pelvic muscles can reduce stress incontinence by 50 to 99 percent. These exercises can build up the muscles in the pelvic floor that manage continence and help you regain bladder control. Here's how to do them:

KEGEL EXERCISES

1) Squeeze in the muscles that you use to hold back urine and to contract your vagina.
2) Hold each contraction for the count of three seconds.
3) Release slowly and relax for three seconds. The release is as important as the squeeze. The goal is muscle function as well as muscle strength.
3) Repeat contractions and release in groups of three many times daily. Try this routine for several days just to get used to it.
4) Increase number of repetitions as you also prolong the amount of time you hold and release, based on a timing that's workable for you—e.g., five times and five seconds. Then if you can, work up to holding for ten seconds with the number of repetitions per day that will fit your own comfort level.
5) Observe your results. Consult with your health advisor as to how many contractions each day may be the control point for you to reach your personal continence goal. However, with biofeedback methods available at some clinics and hospitals, you will

know with greater certainty that you are performing the exercises with the correct muscle groups.

By the way, there's a bonus. Kegel exercises will not only help control urinary problems, but they'll give you the added dividend of increased sexual pleasure. The resulting responsiveness of these muscles can enhance your orgasms.

Collagen therapy has been recently approved by the FDA for stress urinary incontinence. It's a hardy, fibrous, common protein found in our bodies, and it holds tissues and cells together. It is medically used in various therapies when appropriate. Since 3 percent of people tested have an allergic reaction to collagen, a four-week skin test is needed before the procedure is used. Peggy Eastman, writing for the *AARP Bulletin,* explains that "collagen, administered under local anesthesia in a doctor's office, adds bulk to the urethra, thus increasing its resistance to leakage. The procedure is intended for people who've had incontinence for twelve months with no improvement from other therapies [such as Kegel exercises or hormone replacement], and [the patient] should be injected only by doctors who specialize in incontinence."

Liquid intake is more favorable if you drink the major amount of your daily consumption before six o'clock. Then only sip sparingly during the three hours before your bedtime. Also, emptying your bladder every two to three hours is very helpful. Many women tend to hold urine too long for their health and comfort. The less pressure in the bladder, the less stress loss will occur.

Avoid or reduce your consumption of alcohol, caffeine, chocolate, acidic or spicy foods, citrus, tomato juice, and NutraSweet® or any other aspartame sugar-substitutes. All of these can irritate your bladder and compound the intensity of any bladder or urinary tract symptoms.

For managing incontinence until any treatments or exercises are successful, consider this: some of the largest sanitary pad manufacturers are "remarketing" the design of their pads to appeal to women in midlife and older years to protect against accidents from incontinence. Various brands are easily available. You've probably seen them advertised. However, don't let these pads become a crutch. If your incontinence does not need surgical repair, there is a very good chance that the following exercises can be an effective, inexpensive way for you to be worry-free from your problem.

URINARY TRACT INFECTIONS

It's important to recognize that urinary tract infections (UTIs) affect a great number of midlife and older women, causing painful urination as well as the urge to "go" with little or no release of urine. The most common culprit is E. coli bacteria, an organism usually found in the intestinal tract and on the skin surrounding the opening of the vagina. However, in the urinary tract, this bacteria can cause extremely uncomfortable symptoms. In 95 percent of these cases, bacteria are transported from the rectum to the urethra, most often during sexual intercourse or from wiping back to front after bowel movements. These infections can also be caused by tight-fitting pants, panty hose, and activities such as bike riding.

Homeopathic remedies or other alternative treatments can be investigated. On the other hand, if you have severe abdominal cramps with painful urination, you may need a prescription for an antibiotic like Noroxin® from your physician.

Drink lots of water. If you can handle sugar easily, try to consume eight to ten ounces a day of cranberry juice or blueberry juice to keep your bladder lining bacteria-free. These juices are a good preventive measure for women prone to UTI infections.

Dr. Sherie Viencek, in her nutritional counseling practice, recommends freeze-dried cranberry capsules for women who cannot tolerate the high sugar content or calories contained in cranberry juice. Other good prevention techniques for these difficulties are to take extra vitamin C, empty your bladder completely when urinating normally, consider HRT, and be sure to urinate after sexual intercourse to clear the passageway of the urethra from any bacterial residue. Also, it's wise to have a prescription for treatment set aside for traveling, holidays, and weekends, just in case severe infection occurs.

OTHER HEALTH CONCERNS

The health situations mentioned here address only some of the important concerns you need to consider. Too many significant illnesses and emerging conditions are frequently overlooked when diagnosing the over-thirty-five, midlife, and seniorlife woman.

MAJOR HEALTH PROBLEMS

If you know about the following diseases, you can talk about them with your health advisor and inquire about other potential risks.

Thyroid disease affects up to eleven million people and tests should always be part of regular physicals. It can cause significant havoc for midlife women. In certain cases, thyroid complications can eventually lead to grim or even fatal outcomes. Women who have thyroid disease are often misdiagnosed as having depression. Under-active thyroid levels are sometimes associated with high cholesterol levels. *Hypothyroidism: The Unsuspected Illness,* by Broda O. Barnes, M.D. and Lawrence Galton, is an important book about how low thyroid function can affect your body, emotions, and life; basal body temperature described in the glossary is one recommended method for diagnosis; another is having your blood tested for the level of Thyroid Stimulating Hormone.

Clinical depression is suffered by 11.5 million people, two-thirds of them women. Why do only 30 percent of the women who have this problem seek help? The major reasons include social embarrassment, lack of education about the success of various treatments, hopelessness, and isolation. Another barrier to overcome is that many women feel they can work their way through depression with will power, concluding, unfairly, that it's their own fault if they're depressed. Depression may be experienced in repeated episodes throughout one's life or may occur a single time. It's a disease like any other and should be respected as such. Often this ailment is attributed exclusively to psychological causes. A biological dysfunction in the brain or hormonal imbalance, however, often can be the source of depression. Don't ignore any of these possibilities if you are depressed.

Adult Type II diabetes is not an uncommon disease for post-menopausal women. This non-insulin-dependent form of diabetes is strongly linked to an imbalance in sex hormones as well as the presence of an obesity gene. If you aren't sure whether you might be a candidate for diabetes, it is very important to find out. Up to 80 percent of those with adult diabetes are seriously at risk for developing heart disease. Therefore, aggressive prevention or treatment is a must. Medications such as Micronase® or Glucotrol® are used to control this type of diabetes. Consider a customized diet to aid in preventing this illness if your health profile indicates you are at risk—one that does not leave you feeling deprived. Also, maintain a "healthy weight" as explained below.

The American Diabetes Association (ADA) has recently set new guidelines for easier diagnosis. They recommend that everyone should have a fasting plasma glucose at age forty-five—which means nothing to eat eight hours before your blood is drawn. If the results are normal, you should repeat the test every three years thereafter. If your health advisor or you feel you have some risk factors, this test should be taken before you reach forty-five.

Unhealthy body/fat ratio can be a health problem for women at any age. No matter what your weight—low or high—it's crucial to get a body fat analysis. If you have more than a 26 to 30 percent ratio of body fat to total body weight, you need to consider medical, dietary, or exercise intervention—not for vanity or image, but for health. (See the discussion on this subject of weight management at the end of the book.)

Hypertension (high blood pressure disease) is a major health concern. Have check-ups for high blood pressure regularly, because hypertension can lead to strokes and heart attacks. A blood pressure reading of 140/90 or less is considered to be in normal range. Fortunately, it can be controlled; but sadly, almost half of those who have it don't know it. It is especially prevalent in African American women.

Glaucoma refers to a group of eye diseases that cause a buildup of fluid inside the eye. This watery substance forms more rapidly than it can be released, resulting in excessive pressure from within the eye. This pressure can atrophy the optic nerve and damage the retina. It is responsible for half of all adult blindness, affecting mostly those who are over forty.

Glaucoma develops silently with no symptoms. You can only detect it through regular testing and without treatment, it can rob you of your sight. Miotic drugs that reduce the pressure in the eyes or certain surgical procedures can manage the disease quite successfully. Yet after damage has occurred, nothing can be done to restore sight.

Memory difficulties, dementia, and **Alzheimer's** are benefiting from research in the field as never before. Dr. Bruce Wenokur, Medical Director of the Alzheimer's and Memory Impairment Treatment Center in Bloomfield Hills, Michigan (memorydoc@wwnet.com), recommends considering supplements such as phosphatidyl choline, phosphatidyl serine, acetyl L-carnitine, melatonin, DHEA, and ginseng, along with anti-oxidants, coenzyme Q-10, magnesium, amino acids, and Vitamin B complex for better brain function. He has found, for instance, that gingko bilboa, formulated by Murdock from the specific German research standards and sold to the public packaged as Nature's Way®, is producing some marked results with 120 milligram doses for prevention and in mild cases, and with 320 milligrams under more severe circumstances.

Brain Longevity—The Breakthrough Medical Program that Improves Your Mind and Memory, by Dharma Singh Khalsa, M.D., details a plan of action for regenerating concentration, energy, and learning ability as well as treatments for dementia and Alzheimer's. Both he and Dr. Wenokur prescribe, in addition to supplements, estrogen, deprenyl, piracetam, lucidryl, vinpocetine, and hydergine, among others. Obviously, each patient is treated according to individual symptoms and case histories. Any course you want to try personally should be supervised by a qualified practitioner who is knowledgeable in this field.

Difficulties with asthma, allergies, and arthritis can appear before, during, or after menopause, related to various causes and influences, including the changes that come with aging. The treatment for each of these should be explored thoroughly, as new approaches to working with these ailments are always surfacing.

All of these major health concerns, to a greater or lesser degree, are preventable, treatable, even curable. Make certain you tell your health advisor you want to know more about all of them in specific relationship to your health.

PAIN

Chronic pain or periodic pain can come in many forms — headaches, backaches, nerve damage (neurogenic), injuries, arthritis, and psychogenic (not medically identified, but physically experienced)—and can plague us at any age. Don't be surprised if it becomes increasingly prevalent as you grow older. However, newer philosophies about pain management have fortunately surfaced recently, offering more relief without encouraging people to grin and bear it. Women often don't want to admit they are in pain because of embarrassment about not being up to par or past criticism about complaining too much. Research confirms that very few people become addicted to pain medication, and using it when necessary can decrease the intensity and length of the pain cycle in most cases.

DEALING WITH PAIN

MAJOR TYPES OF PAIN

- **Headache:** tension headache, involving contraction of head and neck muscles, or vascular headache, involving changes in the pressure of blood vessels serving the head (including migraines);
- **Lower back pain:** resulting frequently from a combination of changes that come with age, bad posture, infrequent exercise, or excess weight;
- **Cancer pain:** resulting from the pressure of a growing tumor, the movement of tumor cells into other organs, radiation, or chemotherapy;
- **Arthritis pain:** an affliction of the joints, with two common forms: osteoarthritis and rheumatoid arthritis;
- **Neurogenic pain:** not due to past disease or injury, not detectable through signs of damage inside or outside of the nervous system.

NEW TREATMENTS FOR INTERMITTENT OR CHRONIC PAIN

- **Acupuncture:** inserting fine needles under the skin at selected points in the body to release blockages and activate energy flow;
- **Local electrical stimulation:** applying brief pulses of electricity to nerve endings under the skin (e.g., the Alpha-Stim mentioned in the Alternative Treatment Options sections) for pain relief;
- **Brain stimulation:** surgically implanted electrodes are placed in the brain to reduce or eliminate the messages of pain;
- **Drug implants:** pain-relieving medication implanted under the skin for continuous or self-activated dosage.

New and Old Drugs for Pain

- **Aspirin:** interferes with pain signals where they usually originate;
- **Prescription painkillers:** include the opiate-related compounds and usually provide stronger pain relief than aspirin;
- **Antidepressants:** increase the supply of seratonin which cells use as part of a pain-controlling pathway;
- **Antiepilectic drugs:** quiet the distressing pain signals.

Psychological Treatment of Pain

- **Psychotherapy:** to gain insight into the meaning of the pain;
- **Relaxation and meditation therapies:** to relax physical and mental tension that can make any pain worse;
- **Hypnosis:** may lower the pain threshold or the emotional burden of the suffering;
- **Biofeedback:** to learn voluntary control over certain body activities;
- **Behavior modification:** aimed at changing habits, behaviors, and attitudes that can develop in chronic-care patients.

Important Health Tests

The type and frequency of tests to detect various illnesses differ for women in their thirties, forties, fifties, sixties, and beyond. See the "Check-Up Schedule" at the end of this book for details.

Ask your health advisor about these tests and any others that may be important for you:

- Arthritis, allergies, asthma.
- Blood pressure measurement.
- Breast cancer: Mammograms and physician and self-exams.

- Cholesterol levels: HDL, LDL, and triglycerides.
- Colon cancer: Sigmoidoscopy and tests for stool blood.
- Diabetes: Urine screening or fasting plasma glucose test.
- Dual-Energy X-Ray Absorptiometry (DEXA) (measurement for osteoporotic bone loss).
- Fitness/exercise counseling.
- Glaucoma: Eye fluid pressure measurement.
- Heart: EKG; treadmill test if indicated.
- Hormone profiles: FSH, estrogen, progesterone, testosterone (on specific days of the month if menstruating).
- Nutritional Counseling.
- Ovarian cancer screening, if indicated (not often reliable).
- Pap smear.
- Pelvic exam by physician.
- Skin cancer: Physician and self-exams for skin changes.
- Thyroid: TSH (Thyroid Stimulating Hormone).
- Urinary analysis for calcium excretion.

It's rare to meet a woman who is truly eager to make an appointment to take care of nagging but non-acute symptoms. It is even rarer to find a woman motivated to schedule tests for the prevention of potential health problems, which is why you'll find the "Promise Between Friends" contract in Chapter One.

If it were possible to shout something in these pages, it would be: Just do it! It can't be said often enough: The key to good health is prevention. And without our health — well, you know the answer to that one.

CHAPTER SIX

Sexual Sensations, Sensational Sex

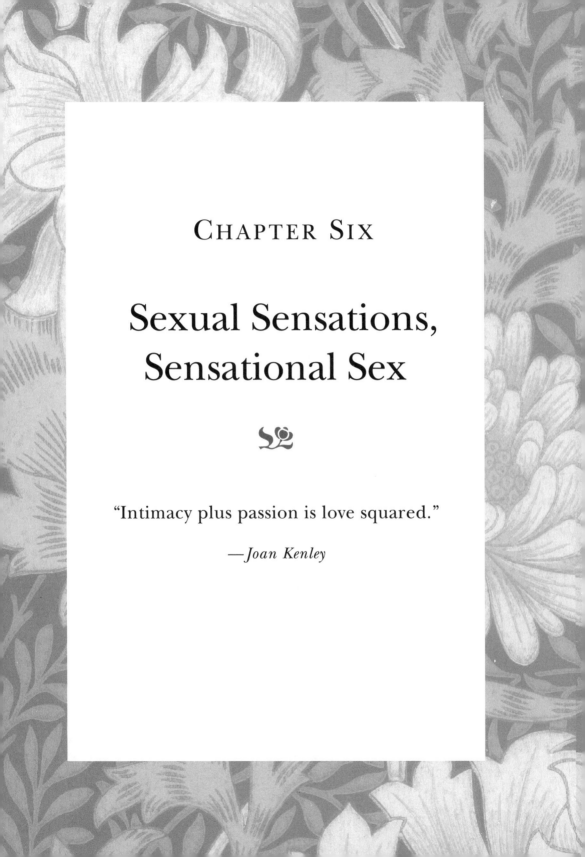

"Intimacy plus passion is love squared."

—*Joan Kenley*

SEXUAL SENSATIONS, SENSATIONAL SEX

Sexuality has always been a "hot" subject. Today it appears that it's hotter than ever for women. Women's magazine covers are screaming about better orgasms and guaranteed climaxes. It is reported that some women find they reach orgasm more easily after thirty-five. Eighty percent of women over sixty report that sex is as good as, or better than, it was in their younger years. Polls claim that two-thirds of the forty-five- to seventy-year-old women in this country are sexually active.

Let's be perfectly clear that healthy sexuality has so many more dimensions than orgasm. Becoming familiar with every part of the subject can encourage greater intimacy, improved relationships, better health for reproductive organs, and, quite possibly, more deeply fulfilling sexual experiences.

What's sad about this subject is that a great number of women are very shy about discussing any concerns regarding the intimate details of their sexual relationships with their health advisors. What's even sadder is that health practitioners often are not educated in a way that qualifies them as experts in sexual matters. Society has prejudices about what "normal" sexual expectations should be for every age group. Hopefully, all of you, regardless of age, will know more about designing a sensual fulfillment program to meet your needs once you have read this chapter.

EMBARRASSMENT ABOUT SEXUAL CONCERNS

There are a great many women who have respectful, trusting relationships with their internists or gynecologists and still prefer to find out about sexual issues elsewhere — but not with friends.

If you are too shy to discuss these issues with those whom you already know, find a knowledgeable professional advisor or resource to educate you about your specific concerns without embarrassment. Consider the numerous sexuality specialists, seminars, and clinics that can address your needs. And there are books, videos, and what you read in this chapter.

Lonnie Barbach, Ph.D., a psychologist, nationally acclaimed author, and expert on sexuality over the last twenty years, has written many books on the subject, including *For Yourself and For Each Other.* The information in this book includes detailed, useful comments on women's sexual information. Lonnie's excellent tapes and videos on the topic of sexuality are referenced for order in her books.

You'll also find sexual information in magazines and on TV/radio talk shows. Look for mail-order ads about sexually informative video tapes for those who are thirty-five-plus. You'll also find books on sexuality at almost every bookstore.

In addition, notices for sexual workshops, lectures, and discussion groups appear on bulletin boards at health practitioners' offices, at dress shops, at gyms, and through on-line computer services. Even if you choose to go to these gatherings and don't feel comfortable talking, you will learn a great deal just by listening.

LOSS OF SEXUAL INTEREST

From the mid-thirties on, women may enter a period of hormone, life, and health changes that can affect sexual passion.

Unpredictable hormone fluctuations can cause unpleasant symptoms—restless nights, mood swings, headaches, fatigue, tender breasts, sexual discomfort, etc.—which can dampen your sexual fires. Your reactions to stress, depression, family conflicts, low energy, or loss of personal closeness with your mate can short-circuit your sexual desire. Experiencing mild to severe health problems can dramatically influence your sexual attitude, response, and responsiveness.

Are you certain you are getting enough hours of deep rest? Remember—if you're experiencing sleeping difficulties, waking up with sweats or other health conditions, you may just be too dog-tired for any sexual activity.

For example, if your problems are related to hormone depletion, estrogen replacement or estrogen-like supplements can improve symptoms, moods, and physical comfort. This, in turn, can enhance libido in general—before, during, or after menopause. Remedies and treatments should address ways to increase blood flow to the pelvis and vagina which can enhance arousal and tissue response. If you're using any kind of estrogen replacement—or any other method—to improve vaginal secretions and not getting the result you want, you may want to adjust your treatment strength or product.

Testosterone and estrogen are the hormones that govern sexual functioning and desire, so you may want to consider a combination regimen of estrogen and testosterone. Additionally, testosterone has been shown to help women feel more energized and more assertive. If you decide to include testosterone supplements in your hormone replacement mix, be sure to consult a doctor familiar with this therapy, beginning with the lowest available dosage to prevent any unwanted side effects.

When it comes to sex and sexuality, the mind-body connection is a very strong one. Taking self-image, self-esteem, health, life situations, and hormones into account can reveal the cause(s) of your loss in sexual interest. After that is determined, then you can feel more confident about exploring how to rekindle your sexual connection.

PAIN DURING SEXUAL INTERCOURSE

You may have real pain during intercourse due to the very real changes in your body. Over time, the vagina may have less moisture and more sensitivity because the vaginal wall tissue can become less resilient, drier, and thinner as you age. Your natural lubricating response to sexual arousal can be diminished by your changing hormones. The pain can send the message to your brain, "Who needs it? Why bother?" Many women stop thinking about sex. Some actively avoid it. Others worry that some major shift, physical or emotional, has occurred.

Of course, you should rule out any serious condition with your health professional. Most likely you're experiencing a normal occurrence. If that's the case, don't be convinced this is a forever situation. In practically every single case of painful intercourse caused by aging and hormone changes, the solutions can be easier than you might imagine.

The most obvious choices to relieve the problem are both lubricants and moisturizers. Each product has a specific use and benefit.

Lubricants are helpful at the time of intercourse, by both the man and woman, to enhance ease and comfort. A lubricant may be all that's needed to make your sexual contact less painful. On the other hand, if your vagina is going through more of a change than diminished sexual secretions, it may not be all you require.

Moisturizers are products that can build up moisture in the vaginal tissues. They are inserted vaginally several times a week, but not at the time of intercourse. Lubricants and/or moisturizers may be sufficient, but if not, there are other proven treatments to enhance vaginal/clitoral tissue and resilience to re-establish natural lubrication. A number of remedies are listed below, along with behavioral suggestions, medications, and various products. If you try something that doesn't work or that you don't like, keep exploring. Review the suggestions. Talk to your doctor. Talk to your friends to see what's working for them. Experiment and enjoy.

Reliable remedies for enhancing your pleasure and relieving discomfort while having sexual intercourse:

Lubricants. Astroglide®, KY Jelly®, and certain aloe vera gels are reliable, non-prescription, water-soluble lubricants that are easily secreted from the vagina after intercourse. They are less likely to promote bacterial growth than oil-based products. You can find them in drugstores and health food stores. Probe® is an excellent product for internal vaginal sexual massage, and it can be found in stores that sell sexual products. Above all, remember this: water-soluble lubricants can be used with latex condoms, but oil-based products, such as coconut oil and the oil from vitamin E suppositories, capsules, or gels, weaken latex condoms. Oil-based lubricants and condoms should never be used together. If your sexual activities don't involve condom use, Vegelatum®, available in health food stores, is a splendidly silky lubricant made by Baby Massage.

Vaginal Moisturizers. Replens® and Gyne-Moisturin® are two reputable brands of water-based vaginal moisturizers you can insert into the vagina every other day to keep your vaginal tissues moist as an aid to making intercourse more comfortable. You may still need a lubricant during sex.

Supplements. Oral zinc sometimes increases vaginal lubrication and secretions. Nutritional specialists recommend a daily dose of 15 to 30 mgs. Foods rich in zinc include wheat germ, oats, nuts, seafood, and meats. Chasteberry, sold as Vitex® in caplet or in tincture form, is recommended for revitalizing vaginal tissue and diminishing pain during intercourse. However, it may take a few months to experience positive results. Black cohosh may bring these same results in four to eight weeks.

Hormone creams, suppositories. Products that contain estrogen can be inserted into the vagina to thicken and rejuvenate vaginal tissue. When applied to the clitoris and surrounding areas, estrogen or testosterone creams can improve sexual response by reversing shrinkage or atrophy. These hormone applications can also relieve dryness and soreness, even decades after menopause. Remember: Don't use any of these hormone creams right before heterosexual intercourse, since your partner doesn't need any of these treatments.

Hormone replacement therapy. Estrogen can increase blood flow to the tissues, increase lubrication, and enhance

your sexual interest. Testosterone therapy can also be helpful to boost your desire and drive.

Estring®. Developed in Sweden and currently available
in the United States, this product, through a vaginal silicone ring, delivers a consistent low dose of estradiol for up
to three months. Estring is a more consistent delivery system than topical vaginal creams, doesn't require constant
applications, and eliminates messiness. It increases lubrication and resilience of the vaginal tissues. The other good
news is that the ring also reduces the urinary urgency that
can occur after giving birth or during midlife and prevents vaginal infections. It does not increase circulating
estrogen, so it is safe for many who ordinarily would not
consider estrogen replacement therapy.

Yeast control. Treatments can curb symptoms and cure
vaginal yeast infections which can interfere with your
sexual desire and comfort. Symptoms can be cottage
cheese–like discharge, burning, itching, and painful
intercourse. Diflucan®, an oral tablet advertised as the
"one-dose cure," is available by prescription and is said to
be comparable to seven days of non-oral medications. It
is sometimes prescribed in conjunction with vaginal
creams. Without a prescription, you can purchase the
following vaginal applications at your drugstore: Week-
long regimens are Gyne-Lotrimin®, Mycelex-7®, and
Monistat-7® as well as the homeopathic remedies such as
Yeast Gard® or Vagisil Yeast Control®; Femstat3® and
Monistat3® are three-day regimens and Vagastat-1® is a single treatment choice. Calendula cream and other topical
products can soothe the area. Important: Don't self-diag-
nose! And don't self-medicate until you've checked with
your medical advisor or nurse practitioner. You may have
something more serious.

Position. If a male/female couple makes love with the woman-on-top position, the woman can control the depth of penetration of her mate's penis and minimize any discomfort that originates from too much penetration.

Antihistamines and decongestants. These, as well as other medications, can cause dryness in the vagina. If it is necessary to use these therapies, drink lots of water and consider using the moisturizing and lubricating suggestions mentioned previously.

Exercise. If you work out regularly, every part of your body will age more gracefully. This concept includes the vagina. Kegel pelvic exercises, described in Chapter Five, will tone the vaginal tissues and surrounding muscles. To improve your sexual responsiveness, begin with a few repetitions several times a day and gradually increase to a number and frequency that brings results. In other words, experiment.

Avoid or limit tight pantyhose; perfumed douches; bath salts; bubble bath; deodorant-treated tampons or panty liners; and harsh soaps, all of which can cause infections, chafing, and rashes.

Odor, Itching, Redness. Products such as Vagisil Feminine Powder® can be used to absorb moisture and to control vaginal odor. If you experience any redness, itching, or dryness, Vagasil Intimate Moisturizer® cream with aloe can be soothing and also help relieve feminine itching and redness.

Urinate after intercourse — always. It helps to clear the urinary tract of any bacteria and prevent infections. Women who are not on estrogen replacement or don't apply topical hormonal creams to the urethra opening and surrounding areas should know that midlife women not on these regimens tend to have more urinary tract infections. The bladder and urethra dry out as estrogen levels drop. These infections are not only unpleasant, but they can wreak havoc with your sex life.

Homeopathic remedies for sexual discomfort include belladonna, lycopodium, and bryonia — but, as always, these treatments should be recommended based on an individual analysis by a homeopathic physician.

Enjoy sexual stimulation and orgasm regularly, with or without a partner, to keep vaginal tissues and surrounding muscles healthy and supple.

Learn about Tantric sexual practices. *Tantra, The Art of Conscious Loving* by Charles and Caroline Muir is an excellent introduction to this exploration of deep sexual pleasure and fulfillment. Caroline and Charles offer seminars on the subject to couples and singles as well as videos and audio tapes. Their business is the Source School of Tantra Yoga in Maui, Hawaii, and they can be contacted for materials and information at 808-572-8364.

Explore deep relationship intimacy. *"Awakening Together"* is a clear, loving book by Martha and Don Rosenthal. It explores how intimacy can disappear in relationships, and offers a powerful step-by-step process to recover lost closeness. The Rosenthals also offer seminars to couples who want to experience these principles with their sensitive and intuitive guidance. To purchase their self-published book or make seminar reservations, you can call them in Vermont at 802-439-6769.

PREGNANCY AND MENOPAUSE

Many women worry about pregnancy through the menopausal years. It is an important concern because your eggs aren't going to wake up singing, "Well, this is it!

Today's the last one!" So you may have irregular periods in the months or years leading up to the actual cutoff. You may believe that the two or three months you haven't had periods indicate that you can't become pregnant. But it's possible that your ovaries haven't stopped releasing eggs yet. Your periods may have stopped temporarily because you are approaching menopause. Or your body may be influenced by stress, strenuous exercise, diet, or medications, any of which can also stop your periods on a temporary basis. If any of these examples apply, it is possible to get pregnant.

Often overlooked are the results of miscarriages for women at any age, including those who are perimenopausal. Perry-Lynn Moffitt's book, *A Silent Sorrow: Pregnancy Loss,* is a sensitive, useful support and resource for women who suffer from this experience.

If your intention is to avoid pregnancy during your transition years, note the rule to remember: If your periods have stopped for twelve months straight, with your health advisor taking other symptoms or indications into the picture, it's safe to say your ovaries are no longer fertile. You can forget about birth control!

CHANGES IN LOVEMAKING SENSATIONS

The "hotspots" that used to be pleasurable and turn your sexual thermostat upward aren't reacting the same way now. Your body is changing and, therefore, your reactions are changing. The places on your body that are pleasure-wired for sexual stimulation are very sensitive, which is why they're called "hotspots" in the first place. Now they're giving you more discomfort or pain than pleasure. Sometimes physical intimacy seems hardly worth the effort.

During menopause, certain body tissues get thinner and

can lose the nice soft cushioning that has protected you from unpleasant sensitivity in the past. So the places that used to turn you on when caressed can now irritate you. Hurt, even. Your partner might be confused because your current reactions are unexpected. Don't be secretive — explain what's happening.

Some women find that estrogen, ginseng, or don quai treatments restore tissues enough to take care of the problem. Others look for new pleasure places. Don't rule out sensual foot massage. Or yummy kisses in the ear.

Like many other things in life, relationships go through changing cycles or seasons. Often your sexual feelings will vary with the seasonal changes going on in your partnership. For example, during the springtimes of your relationship, romance and sexuality are brimming over with life and vigor; in the various summers, urges become hot and passionate; when fall is in the air, the fruits of your relationship can experience deeper intimacy and maturity; if you're dwelling in the winters of your content or discontent, sexuality can slip into a quieter rhythm or even disappear into hibernation—until you arrive at spring again!

The point is to recognize the cycle you are in. Honor it with your partner. When other seasons call, embrace them.

DIFFICULTY REACHING ORGASM

Your changing body may need a change in sexual routine. Everybody needs a certain amount of stimulation to reach climax. Masters and Johnson called it "the orgasmic plateau." Each woman has her own "plateau." At menopause, your blood flow, your nerve connections — all the things that go into making an orgasm — go through estrogen withdrawal. Your "plateau" rises. You need more stimulation to get there. What used to take five or ten minutes can now take much longer.

Since there may be less oxygen and blood going to your muscles, your orgasm could feel weaker than it used to. Estrogen replacement therapy, by improving the condition of your blood vessels and blood flow, can help. Using estrogen, progesterone, or testosterone creams can help. Kegel exercises, described in Chapter Five, can help. There are women who say these "softer, gentler" orgasms are wonderfully pleasurable.

Some women get occasional vaginal spasms, sort of like a charley-horse, during orgasm. The result: Ouch! What's going on? Maybe you're getting too much of the mineral phosphorous. A diet heavy in dairy or soft drinks can cause muscles to react this way. Get some professional advice about what might relieve this. It's possible some magnesium supplements will help.

A final thought: This may be a time for you and your partner to change your ideas about orgasm for a while. It doesn't have to be the Be All and the End All of lovemaking, at least for the moment. Not thinking about orgasm as much could open doors to deeper intimacy between you and your partner. Pay attention to other things, like gentle touching, stroking, and hugging. Perhaps as you learn more about your sexuality, you'll learn more about your orgasms.

DOES YOUR PARTNER UNDERSTAND?

Your mate may be buying into the idea that your changing feelings and biological changes mean saying good-bye to the youthful pleasures of sexuality. He may be harboring the notion that it's "So long, good sex; Hello, zero sex — forever." (Please note that although "he" is used in this section for simplicity, and "she" can be substituted throughout.)

If your partner doesn't know the facts about what you're experiencing, he may feel threatened, leading to sexual uneasiness or withdrawal. Your mate's behavior may be in response to your behavior. What's more, your current responses may trigger fears about his own sexual changes, aging, and mortality. It may be hard for him to face certain truths about his own life. Maybe some of his dreams haven't been realized and some of his hopes may never happen. His ego and sexual interests may be affected by all of these influences. No matter what feelings or behavior your mate has about changes in sexuality and health, menopause, and getting older, it's probably important to plan a good talk. And please remember — timing is everything.

When it comes to communicating about sexuality, experience and maturity can truly be on your side. The sexual urgency and naiveté of your younger years may have given way to openness, self-acceptance, and compassion. Both you and your mate should reflect on your personal needs, even if you're too embarrassed or fearful to express them right away.

Sometimes if you begin with non-verbal expressions of affection, such as holding, touching, and caressing, the words you both want to say may begin to flow more easily. And if talking to your mate is more important to you than he realizes, he needs to know. Well-known books about this subject have helped countless couples communicate in ways they never dreamed possible. There are many women who find that talking stimulates sexual desire. Intimacy that comes with deep personal sharing can be very sexy.

Sexual urges can change as our lives change. One British research study found that men in their late forties and early fifties had less interest in sex than women of the same age. Seventy-five percent of both men and women who are sexually active over age sixty say that sex is better than when they were younger. Because menopause can lead a woman to focus more clearly on her emotional and physical responses, it can result in each partner learning more about each other's sexual satisfaction.

Read to each other from this book. Seek out specialty books, audio tapes, and/or videos on the subject. Find out how this transition can be an exciting journey for both of you.

WHAT WOMEN NEED TO KNOW ABOUT MALE SEXUAL CHANGES

You know you are changing. Do you realize that your partner may be changing too?

"Manopause," male menopause, his midlife crisis — whatever it is, it can truly affect his sex life and sexual responses, whether it's created by hormonal, emotional, or physical causes. What you may want to acknowledge, beyond your own issues, is that he may be experiencing some or all of the following:

- He may take longer to achieve an erection.
- His penis may not be as hard during erections.
- Physical stimulation may be necessary for his penis to achieve erection.
- He may lose his erection during sexual activity.
- His ejaculation may not be as intense, nor as physically urgent as it once might have been.
- Masturbation habits can increase or decrease.
- He may have more anxiety about sexual performance.
- Fights about intimacy, sex, and love can occur more frequently.

- He may have more fantasies about sexual activity with others.
- His desire for sex may be less and he may not feel the need to orgasm.

NEW MEDICATION FOR DIFFICULTIES WITH ERECTION

There is more than an encouraging word here about male impotence. It's a pill called Viagra® made by Pfizer Pharmaceuticals and it may help 60 to 70 percent of the thirty million American men who suffer from difficulties with erection. Since only 5 percent of those who have erectile problems actually seek treatment, women now have the opportunity to urge their mates to consider this non-invasive solution. Methods in the past have involved injections, implants, or mechanical devices that many men have found unworkable or unthinkable.

Pfizer's drug was tested for those who had trouble obtaining or maintaining an erect penis. However, there are physicians in this field who believe that Viagra will make any man's erection last longer. The 100 mg dose can be taken one to four hours in advance of sexual activity, but if there's no turn-on, beware. Arousal is absolutely necessary for an erection. Viagra is a serious drug and should not be misused, overdosed, or passed out casually to friends. Among others, the prevalent side effects are headaches, temporary blue-tinted vision, and lowering of blood pressure.

Researchers predict that the women studies going on now will demonstrate that Viagra can enhance blood flow to the pelvis, an integral part of sexual function but not a guarantee for orgasm. For post-menopausal women, however, estrogen replacement already plays this role, in addition to keeping vaginal tissue healthy and promoting natural lubrication.

Safety Guidelines for Sexual Activity

Women who have not been in the dating scene for a while should be very aware when considering new sexual relationships—especially those who are not yet in menopause. Don't be innocent or regretful about the kind of precautions that are a must if the intention is to become sexually active. Midlife birth control and safe-sex practices should be openly discussed with your physician to prevent unwanted pregnancies or sexually transmitted diseases.

Be on the alert and pay close attention as you read the next section. It contains important information for you and others with whom you'd like to share it.

Any woman at any age engaging in unsafe sexual contact can become infected with AIDS or other sexually transmitted diseases (STDs), also known as venereal disease (VD).

A new love partner can bring a sense of euphoria, urgency, or even carelessness when the heat of the moment strikes. So—Plan Ahead. Most importantly, for encounters with new partners, memorize these rules:

Five Golden Rules for Safe Sex
1) **Limit** your number of sex partners—multiple partners increase the chances for disease.
2) **Discuss** openly and honestly each other's sexual contacts, intravenous drug use, health history, and any blood transfusions prior to 1985, when HIV testing began.
3) **Use only latex condoms** to protect yourself and your

partner from AIDS, which can be transmitted through condoms made from other materials. Know the symptoms and dangers of other sexually transmitted infections as well: chlamydia, genital herpes, genital warts, gonorrhea, hepatitis B, and syphilis. (These are described in the following section.)

4) **Take an HIV test** — both of you — if you intend to have an ongoing, monogamous relationship. In the meantime, use a latex condom for six months or possibly a year after taking the test, even if the results were negative. The virus may be undetectable for as long as twelve months after a person becomes infected.

5) **Practice birth control** if you have any doubt about whether you can still become pregnant.

SEXUALLY TRANSMITTED DISEASES

This information is very, very important to learn if you're sexually active at any age. Many midlife women assume these diseases only happen to teenagers and younger women. Not true. A sexual partner who you feel is trustworthy may have unknowingly contracted a disease or may be a carrier without symptoms, and you might be a carrier yourself. That's why testing and absolute truthfulness are necessary when beginning an intimate relationship with a new partner.

Below, listed alphabetically, are descriptions of the most common sexually transmitted diseases:

AIDS. This is a deadly disease with no cure as of this writing. If you test HIV-positive, always have a second test to confirm the accuracy of the first test. If you are infected, it may take ten to fifteen years for you to develop the full-blown disease. The first signs can be as mild as having the flu with a fever, weight loss, frequent yeast infections, or sweating. AZT and the newer drugs, 3TC and aquinavir, can reduce symptoms and prolong life. The incidence of infection for heterosexual women past forty is 25 percent of the increasingly infected female population of 100,000.

Chlamydia. These non-typical bacterial infections have certain similarities to viruses. The usual symptoms are painful urination or discharge, possible abdominal pain because the urethra is inflamed, or a cervix that is swollen, beefy red and possibly bleeding. Women can develop pelvic inflammatory disease (PID) from chlamydia, and the complications can be infertility or death if left untreated. Unfortunately, there are often no symptoms at all, yet the person infected can still transmit the bacteria to others. Treatment is usually an antibiotic such as tetracycline or clindomycin. Penicillin is not effective.

Genital Herpes. Practitioners and clinics are seeing more and more of this painful viral infection, but since there is no official reporting, the exact numbers are unclear. Symptoms in the genital area are lesions and sores that blister first and then form a crust. In addition to the lesions, swollen glands, muscle aches, fever, painful urination, and vaginal discharge can occur. The initial incidence is usually the most severe. It is most contagious from the time of outbreak to the end of the three-week healing period. It can also be transmitted when there is no visible infection. Acyclovir (sold as Zovirax®) is applied to the infections topically or taken by mouth to relieve symptoms, but at this writing there is no cure. Symptoms may recur every few weeks or never.

Genital Warts. These are very contagious growths that are hard to see or look like flat, fleshy bumps. They are found not only outside, but also inside the vagina as well as the cervix and rectum, making self-diagnosis very difficult. Genital warts are caused by a virus that can easily infect sexual partners. Some forms of this virus can cause cancer of the cervix. Physician examination and Pap smears are essential for a complete diagnosis. The warts can be treated with freezing, laser procedures, electrosurgery, or medication.

Gonorrhea. This is an extremely common, highly contagious disease, affecting more than a million people each year. It is transmitted by vaginal/rectal intercourse or oral-genital sex, and a man can infect others even without ejaculation. Gonorrhea can infect the eyes, inside of the cheek, throat, uretha, rectum, and, most frequently, genital organs. Usually occurring almost immediately within the first ten days of infection, symptoms can include genital burning and swelling, itching, painful urination, an unusual amount of smelly vaginal discharge, and abnormal bleeding. Unfortunately, about half of the women who contract the disease have mild to zero symptoms. Birth control pill users have an almost 100 percent chance of becoming infected if exposed through intercourse. However, pill users are much less likely to develop pelvic inflammatory disease (PID) than non-users, who are at risk for developing tubal scars and loss of fertility. Many other serious complications are also possible. A physician can diagnose this disease by swabbing the secretions of the vagina and cervix to take a gonorrhea culture. Treatment includes either penicillin or antibiotics.

Hepatitis B. This liver disease is also know as serum hepatitis and is a viral infection transmitted mainly through injections with contaminated needles, contaminated blood transfusions, and sexual contact. Without complete recovery, it remains contagious. It can cause cirrhosis or liver cancer. Low energy, nausea, yellowness of the skin, loss of appetite, and fever can be some of the symptoms. There is no known medical prescription that cures this infection. Treatment addresses the symptoms and patients use standard or alternative treatments such as homeopathy for relief. Rest, a healthy diet, and no alcohol are part of the regimen.

Syphilis. Years ago people were ignorant about this disease and subsequently died from it. Today, although syphilis is curable, the symptoms may not be noticed, so you need to know what to look for and self-examine. The first stage is genital lesions or sores—as small as a pinprick up to the size of a dime. There is no pain or itching and the duration is short. The next stage exhibits skin rashes with oozing sores that are highly contagious. A simple blood test can detect the disease and antibiotic treatment can cure it. Most noteworthy, however, is how rapidly the disease can spread without medical treatment, even after the genital sores heal. Syphilis affects the heart, eyes, brain, and other organs. If left untreated, the damage is irreversible.

THE IMPORTANCE OF STAYING SEXUALLY ACTIVE

There is some truth to the idea of "use it or lose it." Your sexual muscles and vaginal tissues are just like the rest of your body—they need to keep in shape. If you have no partner, do it alone. Masturbate. Use dildos, vibrators, your hand. Explore how you can give yourself pleasure as well as lasting sexual health. Some experts recommend that a woman should have at least one orgasm a week to keep everything lubricated and "working."

It may also be time to start thinking creatively with your partner about this new phase of your life. How about trying sensual rather than just sexual encounters — massage, stroking, or cuddling? Or a romantic walk in the woods? Or a great restaurant? Or even a few weeks of planned abstinence to rekindle desire? Or for those of you who want to experiment, have you thought about sexual alternatives to intercourse as an interim or long-term choice? What about music, candlelight, and flowers? Oral sex, mutual masturbation, new erogenous techniques? Should you experiment with sex toys?

If you are interested in experimentation, look at ads in various women's magazines for sexual technique manuals and sexual enjoyment products. In fact, over the last few years, there's been an explosion of female-friendly stores selling female-friendly sexual products. Ask your female friends about one in your city. You might be surprised who knows. Staying user-friendly with your anatomy and your orgasms contributes to a full spectrum of wellness.

Also, certain women turn to finding partners in other arenas in order to have a satisfying sexual experience. There are women at this age who choose to share their sexual intimacy with other women. Still others discover that younger men are the answer for finding sexual fulfillment.

INDIVIDUAL SEXUAL VARIANCES

Every woman is different. You are different from your friends. Your friends are different from their friends. It is true that some women want more sexual experiences after menopause. They feel freer, less afraid of getting pregnant. Maybe their kids have moved out of the house and all of a sudden they feel less inhibited. Maybe they've found a new relationship in midlife or fired up the old one with new spark. Estrogen-like supplements or estrogen replacement can recharge desire. Your sex drive may also increase if you take small doses of testosterone as prescribed by your doctor. Some women also take this "male" sex hormone for more energy. Reflect upon what you want and need for yourself. And don't compare yourself with other women.

WHO'S SEXY ANYWAY?

When we feel sexy, we tend to look and act sexy. When we don't feel sexy, forget it. Yet sometimes women can feel very unsexy, even when others find them quite sensual. Sometimes we feel compromised by the media messages that communicate "sexy" to mean young, thin, smooth, and perky. If you accept too many of those ridiculous messages, your spark can go out. Your ability to flirt back—your sense of your "sexual self"—can suffer. You can become self-conscious. You wonder, "How can anyone be interested in me? I'm so unsexy."

It's time to drum that "sexy equals young or gorgeous" message out of your head. Look around you at seminars or church meetings or department stores. Look at "older" women with sexual magnetism or beauty not represented by the media. What do they have in common? They're confident. They know that sexiness is an attitude. A healthy spark can light a fire at any age.

CHAPTER SEVEN

Beating the Odds— Heart Disease, Cancer, and Osteoporosis

"In facing the facts and embracing
the fear, we travel on hidden roads
that reveal our destiny. May grace
be our companion."

—*Joan Kenley*

HEART DISEASE, CANCER, AND OSTEOPOROSIS: AN OVERVIEW

❧

A word of warning: This chapter is full of important information and suggestions. Take it in *slowly*. The intention is to cut through the confusion of complex subjects and give you an overall balanced picture. Don't get "information over-load." It may make sense to digest one subject at a time. Or to just read it through lightly the first time and reread it later for more detail. Understanding will come more easily at a pace you find comfortable.

Heart disease, cancer, and osteoporosis are the top three silent thieves of women's midlife health. They are the major silent killers of women from ages sixty-two to eighty. These serious illnesses don't scream out at you like hot flashes and sweats. You can't feel or see them like mood swings and fatigue. In many cases, there's no indication that something is amiss until you have a medical crisis. If you follow the prevention guidelines presented in these pages, these silent spoilers may have less of an opportunity to visit your doorstep. Also, no one should forget the life-saving value of routine testing for early detection and treatment of major illnesses. Midlife women can expect to live to age eighty and possibly longer. The quality of these later years becomes more and more important. Each woman has two health alternatives: pay attention in your early years, or pay the price later on.

Preventing serious illness is always the best choice, but let's acknowledge that prevention is often difficult. Far too many times, it takes a serious health scare to convince people to take action.

Dr. Dean Ornish, President/Director of the Preventive Medicine Institute in Sausalito, California, and author of *Reversing Heart Disease,* says, ". . . I think it is very difficult to motivate people to follow a diet or to stop smoking or to engage in other desirable behaviors. . . . Telling somebody that they may live longer if they just eat less meat or stop smoking is not terribly motivating." Some people have emotional or situational issues connected to the habits they have. On the other hand, there are those with no major underlying problems who still have biological cravings for such things as smoking, chocolate and certain other foods, and drugs.

This biology-versus-behavior consideration is extremely relevant for midlife women as they deal with the physical and emotional changes thrust upon them during "The Change." It's important for you to contemplate what relates to your habits, cravings, and addictions at this point as well as how those issues affect later life. Is it the biology of your hormones that determines whether you care about choosing a healthy lifestyle? Is it your denial that you could become seriously ill? Or is it your inertia that tells you it's not worth it to bother changing your life around because you have some psychological wounds to heal? Examine your issues, moods, attitudes, and motivations when you answer these questions. Explore how you can pursue the healthy rewards you deserve.

If you or someone you love has to face the reality of serious illness, it will take courage, strength, and deep personal questing to meet this challenge with the most positive and pro-active frame of mind. Inside your family circle or with a support group of others in a like situation, whether you are the patient or the caregiver, you need to seek a network of alliances for emotional, physical, and spiritual healing. There are a variety of books on the subject of facing illness and dying, and one of the most poignant is Dr. Jean Shinoda Bolen's *Close to the Bone—Life-Threatening Illness and the Search for Meaning.*

THE FACTS

Heart disease is the number one killer of American women. One out of every nine women between the ages of forty-five and sixty-four has heart disease, and the percentage of those over age sixty-five among these is one in three. Each year, more than 500,000 women in the US die of heart disease, heart attacks, strokes, and blood vessel diseases. The majority of these are Caucasian and African-American. Cardiovascular diseases are also the leading cause of disability for women. Twice as many adult women die of heart and blood vessel diseases than die of all forms of cancer.

Breast cancer is the most feared cancer, yet it is one of the most curable when detected early. The emotions surrounding breast cancer as opposed to other serious cancers seem to cause more misinformation. Fortunately, there is promising research to more easily and effectively obtain early diagnosis for this terrible disease. For African-American women, breast cancer is the number one cause of cancer mortality, yet it does not come close to the number of deaths caused in this group by heart disease and hypertension. Lung cancer, caused almost entirely by smoking, ranks first as the cancer killer for women of all other ethnic groups, with 59,000 deaths yearly. Breast cancer mortality was down in 1994 for the first time in ten years, to 41,400. Colon cancer is responsible for the demise of 25,000 women annually.

Osteoporosis is another considerable health threat. Almost 50 percent of all women over fifty will develop fractures from osteoporosis. It is a disease causing loss of bone mass in the skeleton of the body, resulting in bone fractures from a sudden movement, strain, bump, or fall. The National Osteoporosis Foundation reports that deaths from causes related to osteoporosis number about 50,000 yearly, mostly women. Few know that osteoporosis affects twenty million American women, causing 1.3 million fractures annually, at a yearly cost of seven to ten billion dollars.

IMPORTANCE OF FAMILY HEALTH HISTORY

Your genes give you certain traits, which may include tendencies to get certain diseases. Did your mother have trouble with her periods? Did she have an early menopause? A difficult or an easy one? Did your grandmother have osteoporosis? Did your grandparents live happily to a ripe old age? That's family health history. Knowing it gives you important information about yourself and about how to protect your health. Some tendencies toward high blood pressure, alcoholism, being overweight or underweight, or having a weak immune system are related to family health patterns. We can also inherit the risk of having osteoporosis, diabetes, heart disease, obesity, and certain kinds of cancer.

An inherited tendency is not a bad or a dangerous thing in and of itself. Think of it as a gift, a signpost for you to pay attention, a tool for you to know about and to use. It's not a guarantee of illness. Talk to your family first — your parents, grandparents, siblings. Know more. There are specialists called medical geneticists who can help you determine and interpret the risk of contracting diseases that are prevalent in your family.

HEART DISEASE

Is there incidence of heart disease, stroke, high cholesterol, high blood pressure, or diabetes in your family? Did any of the women have early menopause in their late thirties or early forties? If your answer to any of these questions is yes, it's possible you may have inherited certain risk factors for cardiovascular problems. Unfortunately, just getting older increases your chances of getting heart disease. Fortunately, the proven facts are that a heart-healthy lifestyle and preventive measures can work wonders to keep your precious heart in good shape.

HEART DISEASE IN WOMEN

Relatively few women are aware of the dangers of heart disease, strokes, and other cardiovascular disorders. These conditions just aren't high on their list of health concerns. They should be. The American College of Cardiology reported in 1993 that women at any age are more likely than men to die after a heart attack. Dr. Philip Greenland,

Chief of Preventive Medicine at Northwestern Medical School, reports that both heart attack and stroke deaths in females have exceeded male deaths since 1984.

All cardiovascular diseases combined cause more than half a million deaths among women each year. Heart problems are often thought of as a "man's disease," but that belief has been shown to be a myth. It is true that research on heart disease has been done almost exclusively on middle-aged and middle-class men. However, that is about to change with the National Institute of Health directing the Women's Health Initiative to study heart disease as well as osteoporosis and cancer. It is also true that women at menopause and after are more at risk for heart disease than pre-menopausal women, who have built-in protection from their estrogen supply. Estrogen helps blood vessels stay open and promotes good circulation. Keep in mind that heart attacks are the number one cause of death among post-menopausal women.

Saralyn Mark, M.D., endocrinologist and Medical Advisor for the Office on Women's Health, U.S. Department of Health & Human Services, Washington, DC, tells us that "women do not do as well as men after heart disease is diagnosed. Within a year after a serious heart attack, women have a 45 percent mortality as compared to 10 percent for men. Overall, heart disease accounts for a greater proportion of all deaths in women (52 percent) than in men (46 percent)."

Some sobering statistics from the American Heart Association: Over fifty-five million men and women have one or more forms of cardiovascular disease. (Women represent most of those with high blood pressure and half of those with the remaining disorders.)

1) High blood pressure — 65 million

2) Coronary heart disease — 6.3 million
3) Stroke — 3 million
4) Rheumatic heart disease — 1.3 million

WOMEN'S HEART DISEASE SYMPTOMS

Symptoms for heart disease are harder to detect in women. Partly because female hormonal changes tend to cause data variations, women haven't been part of major heart studies in the past. More recently, however, the HERS Research Project has helped by studying the relationship of heart problems and hormone replacement therapy in post-menopausal women with existing heart disease. Kathy Berra, clinical coordinator at the HERS Stanford site, tells us of another consideration: "Prior to menopause, women rarely develop heart disease. However, diabetic women often develop heart disease in their forties and fifties, and it's often missed as a diagnosis. Also, women generally develop heart disease ten to fifteen years after menopause."

Dr. Saralyn Mark reminds us that heart disease diagnosis through stress tests "are not as accurate in women. When compared to men, there is both a higher false positive rate in young women who do not have coronary artery disease and a higher false negative rate in older women with true disease. Recent studies reveal that exercise echocardiography may enhance our ability to detect heart disease in women."

There is some unfortunate news from recent studies: women who have heart disease symptoms often do not seek medical help. Furthermore, there are women who have gone to hospitals or doctors' offices complaining of chest pain who have not been taken seriously. Many health professionals still believe the myth that heart disease is a man's disease. Appropriate tests are not given to women as readily or as often. Women with a pain in their jaw, nausea, or shortness of breath may be having a heart attack. But because they don't have the classic "elephant sitting on the chest" male symptom, they may be told they have heartburn, indigestion, or anxiety, without receiving a careful examination for cardiac distress.

To add insult to injury, research has found that women dressed in conservative suits found their complaints taken more seriously than casually dressed female patients.

If a woman acts desperate or emotional or cries too much about her pain, surveys have found that she is considered to be high-strung and hysterical by certain physicians and is offered tranquilizers, sleeping pills, sedatives, or a visit to a psychiatrist. In order to protect yourself, it's good to know these facts. On the other hand, this is definitely not the case in all circumstances.

SIGNS OF HEART ATTACK OR STROKE

Symptoms of a heart attack include:
- faintness;
- shortness of breath;
- back pain that leads to deep pulsing or aching in the right bicep;
- chest pain or a sensation of chest tightening that lasts for more than fifteen minutes;
- severe discomfort, pain, banding, tightness, heaviness or pressure in the jaw, neck, shoulder, arm; pressure between the breasts, in the neck, jaw, shoulders, between the shoulder blades, or down either arm ;
- nausea and vomiting if associated with above symptoms; and

HEART

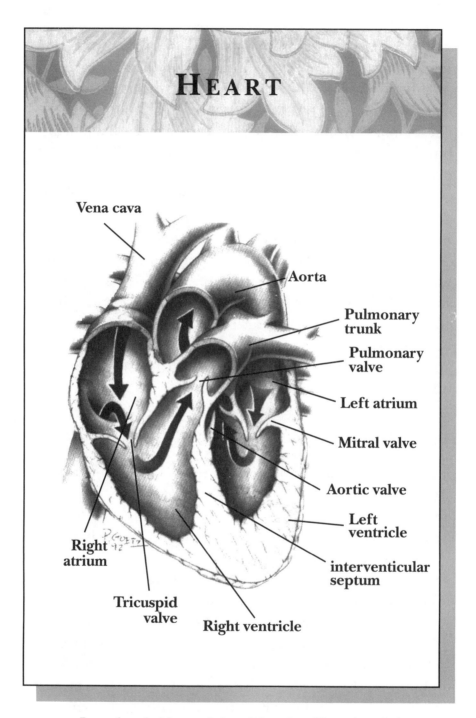

Vena cava

Aorta

Pulmonary trunk

Pulmonary valve

Left atrium

Mitral valve

Aortic valve

Left ventricle

interventicular septum

Right atrium

Tricuspid valve

Right ventricle

Reproduced with permission: ©American Heart Association;
Heart and Stroke Facts, '92—94.

- profound sweating, with the other symptoms mentioned.

Symptoms of a stroke include:

- impaired speech or problems understanding speech;
- sudden severe dizziness or headaches;
- dimming of vision or loss of sight; and
- sudden numbness, weakness on one side of your body, i.e., the loss of strength in one leg or arm.

DECREASING YOUR RISK OF HEART DISEASE

You can't just swallow something to prevent heart disease, but you can greatly reduce your risk. Begin by trying to face any resistance you may have to becoming heart-wise. If you have any hesitations, examine why you might want to reject changing your lifestyle. Work with yourself. Then give yourself time, patience, and self-love to adjust to a heart-healthy life program. Know what can be treated or improved:

High blood pressure. 140/90 or above is cause for concern. If your first reading is high, you will need to have your blood pressure taken two more times on two different days to confirm the diagnosis.

High blood cholesterol. Many health guidelines consider a total cholesterol count over 240 a risk factor for cardiovascular disease. From that information, would you conclude that a reading of 285 would be better than a total cholesterol of 235? Probably not.

The total cholesterol reading includes the positive HDL numbers and the harmful LDL count. The point, of course, is that the total cholesterol numbers mean nothing without knowing the HDL ratio to the overall count. When we look at it from that perspective and realize that the woman with 285 has a 4.4 ratio with a 65 HDL, it's another story, particularly when we also know that the woman with 235 has a 38 level of HDL and a ratio of 6.2, which is not good. Any ratio of HDL to total cholesterol higher than 4.5 can be considered a potential risk factor for heart disease.

Diabetes. Adult Type II (the type of diabetes that requires diet, exercise, and sometimes oral medications as compared to Type I, which requires insulin shots) happens particularly in midlife women carrying an excess of upper body weight. A woman with Adult Type II diabetes is three times more likely to get heart disease than a Type II diabetic man. It's extremely important to have your blood glucose levels checked because you may not notice symptoms for many years. Not many women realize that 80 percent of those who have this kind of diabetes will die of some form of heart or blood vessel disease.

High triglycerides. The 300 to 500 range can be dangerous if your LDL cholesterol is also high, along with a low HDL cholesterol. Obesity adds risk to this picture. Triglycerides below 150 mg/dl is considered the optimal level, yet those with no other risk factors can have a reading of 300 that is not considered to be a problem.

Dangerous Behaviors for Heart Health

Smoking. The carbon monoxide in cigarettes is the same chemical that comes out of your car's exhaust pipe. It limits the oxygen going to your heart, damages your arteries, can raise your cholesterol level, and increases the chance of blood clots. It can also bring on menopause one to two years early. It's the worst thing a woman can do. Some experts say that two years after quitting cigarettes, your chances of getting heart disease go down by half.

Fatty foods. The high cholesterol content of saturated fat in meat, high-fat dairy products, lard, and butter, as well as hydrogenated vegetable fats like palm oil and coconut oil, clog arteries and lead to heart attacks. When choosing your oils for cooking, condiments, or dressings, choose wisely from this list: canola, corn, flax (don't heat this one), olive, peanut, safflower, soybean, or sunflower seed. Remember too, that high-fat foods — with fat of any type — tend to make you gain weight. Your fat intake for good health should range between 20 and 30 percent of your total daily calories.

Obesity. The body stress and heart-risk factors caused by obesity are a big contributor to heart disease, particularly if your body weight composition is over 30 percent fat. This percentage is more important than the total pounds you weigh because it is a more accurate health indicator. Weight distribution is also a key risk factor. If you carry more weight in your stomach and lower belly, a weight pattern more common to men, you are more at risk for heart disease. Women with heavier hips and thighs are luckier in this case. Finding the right diet for your body and your lifestyle can be a challenge, but the pay-off is great. Keep a list of everything you eat for a week to truly understand what you're consuming. Find a weight management consultant who can address your particular body type and individual food choices. The aim is to focus on total wellness, not weight loss alone. Read the last section in this guidebook on "Weight Issues."

Heavy alcohol consumption. If your alcohol intake is interfering with your life or your health but seems too difficult to handle yourself, seek out professional counseling, clinics, support groups, or programs to help you. Alcohol can destroy your liver and certain brain functions while increasing bone loss and your chances of colon cancer. It also raises your risk of breast cancer. In moderation, alcohol can be heart protective, but if heavy use is a problem, only you can determine what will motivate you to take action.

HEART-HEALTHY BEHAVIOR

Reduce stress even if you seem to thrive on it—emotional stress, stressful schedules, negative pressures, and sometimes even positive excitement can be harmful to your heart. Dr. John Arpels reminds us that even though "stress in and of itself probably doesn't cause disease, it is the effect stress has on our lifestyle or on our immune system that creates problems. It especially decreases the available estrogen in the system." A stressful schedule often leads to poor nutritional habits, inadequate time to exercise, and excessive use of caffeine and alcohol, not to mention poor sleep.

Exercise at least three times a week if you aren't currently working out that regularly. But first be sure to have clearance from your health advisor to confirm that your current health and physical condition would not limit your range of exercise choices. Start a moderate program you can build on — one that suits your age and individual physical requirements. Just walking twenty to thirty minutes three to five times a week is helpful to your heart. If you can, develop a regimen that is mapped out by a personal fitness instructor at your local gym, health club, or clinic. Or use a reputable, reasonable video.

Do you drive each time you go out instead of walking or biking? A non-active lifestyle invites heart disease. Regular exercise helps lower blood pressure and stimulate the formation of new bone. It burns fat. It can raise the "good cholesterol" in your body and lower the "bad." It reduces stress. And besides, it makes you feel better. Plan to exercise before 8:00 p.m. to avoid insomnia from over-activity.

Eat heartfully by consuming no more than 30 percent fat in your diet, keeping animal and dairy fat only a small portion of that percentage. Keep your regimen full of grains, fruits, and vegetables. Use fish, poultry, and soy products to fulfill protein requirements. Limit red meat consumption.

PREVENTION METHODS AND BENEFITS

Vitamins C, E, B6, Psyllium, and Folic Acid can be heart-healthy additions to a heart-wise eating program. But first check dosage with your practitioner.

A low-dose aspirin regimen is controversial, but it is a heart protection practice some men have been using for years. One recent major Nurses Health Study showed that women were able to prevent heart attacks by taking one to six low-dose aspirin tablets weekly or 60 mgs every three days. With this evidence, women concerned about heart disease are considering aspirin regimens. However, some experts disagree about this one.

Studies show that estrogen replacement for menopausal and post-menopausal women or those who have had their ovaries removed is a major prevention for heart disease because it helps to maintain a healthier blood flow throughout the system. Studies of post-menopausal women found that those taking estrogen for five years or more had a mortality rate from heart disease that was 40 percent lower than women the same age who were not on hormone therapy. Some women feel this protection against heart disease outweighs their own personal concerns about breast cancer. Others do not.

BREAST CANCER

❧

Controversy abounds about the very emotional subject of breast cancer. Other cancers are more deadly and affect greater numbers, but this area of our bodies has so much meaning, symbolism, and physical sensitivity that it's almost impossible to remain objective or hopeful when breast cancer is diagnosed. The causes of this cancer are not clearly identifiable. The debate continues and misinformation abounds. The intent of this chapter is to present guidelines that will influence a balanced view of the situation as it currently exists.

CONTROVERSY ABOUT ERT AND BREAST CANCER

The relationship between breast cancer and estrogen replacement therapy needs to be examined. Too frequently what we hear or read is tinged with bias or fear or incomplete information. Try not to be reactive. Be educated. Then choose for yourself what to believe.

There have been ten reports with evidence that women who were on hormone replacement therapy when their breast cancer was detected lived longer than the women not on hormones. Some speculate this outcome may be the result of the close medical monitoring these patients received because of their combined breast cancer care and ERT/HRT regimen. Others speculate that it is because of the known enhancement to the immune system which estrogen provides, as well as the anti-metastasis properties promoted by estrogen.

However, if you have an estrogen-dependent tumor, estrogen may increase the rate of growth. In general conversation and media reports, this dynamic often translates into claims that hormone replacement "causes breast cancer." That linkage is not fact-based as of this writing.

Projections of twenty years of hormone use and its breast cancer risks have been reported recently. In September of 1995, two apparently contradictory studies about this hormone/breast cancer debate appeared in two respected medical journals. It was stated in one study that taking hormones for twenty years would cause women a 50 percent increase in the risk of breast cancer. The other said extended use of estrogen caused no significant risk. The bottom line is that you had to understand the way the information was presented. Many thought the first report meant that 50 percent of the women taking hormones were at risk for getting breast cancer. They didn't realize that the percentage reflected an increase of risk to about 3 percent, as opposed to the previously assumed risk factor of around 2 percent.

The Women's Health Digest, published by the founder of the National Menopause Foundation, Morris Notelovitz, M.D., Ph.D., printed an article by Barry Wren, M.D., that clarified the results:

- For every one hundred women past age fifty not taking HRT and living to age seventy, six have a relative risk for breast cancer.
- For every one hundred women past age fifty taking HRT and living to age seventy, nine have a relative risk for breast cancer.

From another point of view, there are those who have concluded that women are being used as guinea pigs, because the cause and effect of hormones — estrogen and progestin or progesterone — and breast cancer remains controversial. Any chosen path can have 30 to 40 percent placebo effect, so it is important to believe in both your treatment and your practitioner.

You also must decide if the benefits of estrogen in reducing death from heart disease and the incidence of osteoporosis and colon cancer should be a personal consideration. Clinical studies regarding hormones and breast cancer are now under way to present more long-term information, but those reports aren't scheduled for release until 2004 and 2010.

FACTS: ESTROGEN AND BREAST CANCER

Doctors usually do not prescribe estrogen for women who have had breast cancer, particularly estrogen-dependent cancers. That's because, although estrogen doesn't cause normal breast cells to turn into cancer cells, estrogen may cause some already cancerous cells to grow faster. So most doctors choose not to prescribe estrogen at all.

For those women who have had breast cancer and want to take estrogen, Dr. Arpels tells us, "There are many menopause experts both here and abroad who feel strongly that giving hormone replacement to these women will have no impact one way or another on the natural history of their breast cancer." Some studies have compared women who have been treated for breast cancer and then used hormone replacement therapy with those who did not. There were no statistically significant results indicating that hormone users had a greater risk of breast cancer recurrence or death from the cancer than did non-users.

In addition, Arpels reports, "a number of studies show that were breast cancer to develop, those women who are on hormone replacement at the time of its detection have a better survival rate than if they had not been on hormones. This goes along with data which suggests that the immune system may be enhanced by the estrogen, which also lowers the rate of mestastatic breast disease — the spread of cancer that is so dangerous."

Based on all the breast cancer/hormone controversies, many women are afraid to try hormone replacement. However, if a woman's menopausal symptoms are so harsh that her life is miserable and no alternative choices for relief seem to help, she may decide to take hormone therapy for just a few years to improve the quality of her life during the rough transition.

Estriol is a weak estrogen produced by the placenta, and it can be compounded and given to those who have or have had breast cancer. For some, it helps reduce various menopausal symptoms. Dr. Henry Lemon conducted a study showing that 2.5 to 15 mgs per day could remit or arrest breast cancer in over one-third of his patients while causing few or no side effects.

You need to choose an option you feel comfortable using. If, after learning the facts, you are worried that hormone therapy will increase your risk of breast cancer, then hormone replacement may not be the best choice for you. SERMs, the "designer" estrogens, and plant estrogens such as soy and red clover are described in the chapter on hormones and may be worth considering. Other alternative therapies are described throughout the book.

For hot flashes, 400 units of d alpha-tocopherol vitamin E and/or 200 mgs of B6 twice a day along with a low fat, high complex carbohydrate diet is recommended. Soybean products and other plant estrogen foods, botanical tinctures, herb teas, etc., may be suggested. Relaxation, meditation, slow breathing techniques, and exercise can offer relief. You can explore homeopathic remedies, acupuncture, Ayurvedic, treatments or any other complementary treatments that you find helpful in your community. There's more on hot flashes in Chapter Five.

INCREASED RISKS OF BREAST CANCER WITH AGE

You may have heard that breast cancer strikes one in nine American women, but that refers to each woman's lifetime probability if she reaches age 110. If you're over fifty, your risk increases in the following way:

The National Cancer Institute reports that from age fifty to fifty-nine, a woman's risk factor is around 2 percent. Over the next decade, it can increase to 3 or 4 percent with the peak years falling between sixty-four and sixty-eight. Over age seventy, the risk can be 5 percent or more. Recent studies point to breast cancer possibly being caused by a mix of abnormal genes, environment, and lifestyle. Exactly what the mix is not clear. But truthfully, the jury is still out. Nobody is sure what causes breast cancer. It occurs in younger women as well as those over fifty. Fortunately, the statistics show death rates are decreasing and longevity increasing for the 182,000 women developing breast cancer each year.

WOMEN AT RISK FOR BREAST CANCER

Risk factors are red flags, not pre-determined outcomes. You need to be aware. You need to pay attention. Know the warning signs. Doctors use "risk" to describe certain traits, lifestyle habits, or conditions that tend to give you a greater statistical chance of getting certain diseases. While the

LONG-TERM ERT RELATIVE RISK AFTER 50

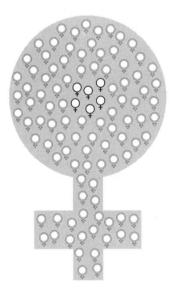

Indicates *relative risk,* not *absolute risk,* for those not taking HRT after age 50

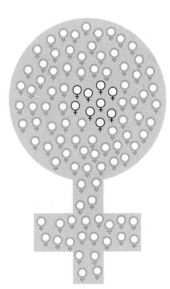

Indicates *relative risk,* not *absolute risk,* from long-term use of HRT after age 50

Source: Barry Wren, M.D., in *The Women's Health Digest*
Design: Roland Gauthier

causes of breast cancer remain unclear, some patterns have emerged.

It's important to know that "risk" doesn't mean "cause." It doesn't mean you will get a disease. But if you have a mother and sister or two sisters who have had breast cancer, don't panic: less than 15 percent of the women with breast cancer have a close relative with the disease. So here's what risk really means: you not only should take note, but certainly take steps to take charge of your health and change what can be changed.

Two-thirds of the women who get breast cancer don't have any risk factors, but it is important to know what they are.

Women have risk factors if:
• they started their periods before age twelve;
• they entered menopause after fifty-five;
• they're older than forty, and especially older than fifty;
• their mother and sister(s) have had breast cancer;
• they've never had children;
• they've had their children late in life;
• they eat a lot of fat;
• they smoke;
• they don't exercise;
• they have more than two alcoholic drinks daily; and
• they're overweight.

Educate yourself further about your own risk by getting a formal Breast Cancer Risk Analysis from a breast clinic or, if indicated, see a medical geneticist.

Please review the following pages carefully.

Breast Changes to Look For

The American Cancer Society lists the following breast changes — if they persist — as warning signals:
- lump(s);
- skin irritation;
- swelling;
- tender nipples;
- nipple discharge;
- nipple retraction; and
- scaliness or dimpling.

Many of these symptoms are also associated with fibrocystic disease, a general term for all non-cancerous conditions that can cause tenderness and lumps. Four out of five lumps that are detected are not cancerous. Yet some non-cancerous lumps can become malignant if they are not removed. A skilled gynecologist or breast specialist should examine any changes in your breasts.

Early Detection of Breast Cancer

For all women, for the moment, no matter what their "risk factors," the American Cancer Society tells us that the best breast cancer "prevention" is early detection through mammograms.

Mammograms can spot 90 percent of breast cancers when they are in their earliest, treatable, curable stages up to two years before a lump can be detected in a self-exam or by your physician's breast exam.

There are two types of mammograms:
1) Screening for women with no symptoms.
2) Comprehensive/Diagnostic, for women of any age

who have lumps or any symptoms of breast cancer such as the ones just mentioned. Future tests such as digital screening and ultrasound eventually will reveal even more as the technologies improve.

The other important method of detection is monthly self-exams. You may be surprised to know that women who are self-examining discover 85 percent of breast lumps through this method. Sad to say, however, as women become older, they are less likely to self-examine—just when they are at their highest risk. Breast self-exams have found tumors that were undetected by mammograms, so always do your monthly self-exams. Women should begin self-exams when they are in their twenties and develop it into an art by forty. And remember, it's wise for everyone to have an annual breast exam by a physician.

Get advice on how to give yourself breast exams that really count. Cancer associations, breast clinics, and your physician can give you demonstrations and brochures to educate you about the best procedures.

Once you make this commitment, it's easier to remember if you mark your calendar or just decide it's the same day each month. Then put up some reminders until you get into the habit. Also revisit the diagrams and self-exam techniques from time to time.

MAMMOGRAM FREQUENCY

Even though mammogram screening is controversial, there are guidelines to consider:

A baseline mammogram should be performed between the ages of thirty-five and forty unless otherwise indicated. This test will provide a reference point for later evaluations. The American Cancer Society and the National Cancer

Institute, as well as eleven other reputable medical organizations, currently recommend having a mammogram at least every one or two years between the ages of forty and forty-nine, and each year after age fifty.

There is debate within the medical community about the necessity of this frequency between the ages of forty and fifty. Similarly, there are some health providers that believe yearly mammograms after you're fifty is too often. Data reported from Scandinavia shows the need for screening every twelve to eighteen months for those between forty-five and fifty-five. These tests reportedly can lower the death rate from breast cancer because there is particularly rapid tumor growth in this age group. Certainly it can be unsettling to have the experts at odds. An important part of your individual health regimen is to be educated about choices when the experts disagree. Then be comfortable with your personal mammogram screening schedule.

APPROVED GUIDELINES FOR MAMMOGRAMS

- The imaging center should be accredited by the American College of Radiology and meet federal guidelines and standards for equipment, personnel, and timely reporting of results. To find out if your center is certified or to find one that is, call 800-4-CANCER.
- Request that a registered technician perform your mammogram. Ask for credentials.
- Only two to three films of each breast should be taken to limit total radiation. However, more may be needed to verify questionable areas.
- Ask for verification that the equipment is used only

Breast Self-Examination

Breast self-examination (BSE) should be done once a month so you become familiar with the usual appearance and feel of your breasts. Familiarity makes it easier to notice any changes in the breast from one month to another. Early discovery of any change from what is normal is the main idea behind BSE. The recovery outlook is much better if you can detect breast cancer in the early stage.

If you menstruate, the best time to do BSE is 2 or 3 days after your period ends, when your breasts are least likely to be tender or swollen.

If you no longer menstruate, pick a day—such as the first day of the month—to remind yourself. The following pages show you how to examine your breasts.

Source: American Cancer Society.

Tumor Size and Detection Chart

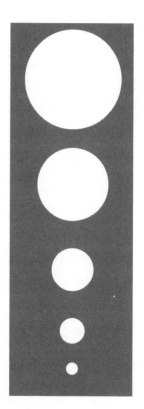

Average-size lump found with untrained self-exam.

Average-size lump found with occasional self-exam.

Average-size lump found with monthly self-exams.

Average-size lump found with first mammogram.

Average-size lump found with regular mammograms.

Source: The Breast Health Program of New York. Adapted by Roland Gauthier.

BREAST SELF-EXAM

Breast self-examination (BSE) should be done once a month so you become familiar with the usual appearance and feel of your breasts. Familiarity makes it easier to notice any changes in the breast from one month to another. Early discovery of any change from what is normal is the main idea behind BSE. The recovery outlook is much better if you can detect breast cancer in the early stage.

If you menstruate, the best time to do BSE are days seven to nine of your monthly cycle, when your breasts are least likely to be tender or swollen.

If you no longer menstruate, pick a day—such as the first day of the month—to remind yourself. The following pages show you how to exam your breasts.

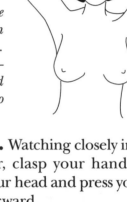

2. Watching closely in the mirror, clasp your hands behind your head and press your hands forward.

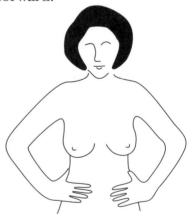

1. Stand before a mirror. Inspect both breasts for anything unusual such as any discharge from the nipples, puckering, dimpling, or scaling of the skin.

The next two steps are designed to emphasize any change in the shape or contour of your breasts. As you do them, you should be able to feel your chest muscles tighten.

3. Next, press your hands firmly on your hips and bow slightly toward the mirror as you pull your shoulders and elbows forward.

158

Some women do the next two steps of the exam in the shower because fingers glide over soapy skin, as well as making it easy to concentrate on the texture underneath.

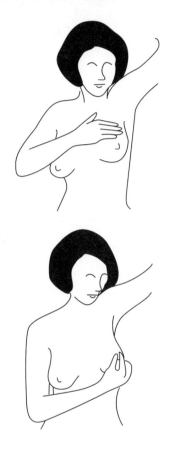

4. Raise your left arm. Use three or four fingers of your right hand to explore your left breast firmly, carefully, and thoroughly. Beginning at the outer edges, press the flat part of your fingers in small circles, moving the circles slowly around the breast. Gradually work toward the nipple. Be sure to cover the entire breast. Pay special attention to the area between the breast and the underarm, including the underarm itself. Feel for any unusual lump or mass under the skin.

5. Gently squeeze the nipple and look for a discharge. (If you have any discharge during the month—whether or not it is during BSE—see your doctor.) Repeat steps 4 and 5 on your right breast.

6. Steps 4 and 5 should be repeated lying down. Lie flat on your back with your left arm over your head and a pillow or folded towel under your left shoulder. This position flattens the breast and makes it easier to examine. Use the same circular motion described earlier. Repeat the exam on your right breast.

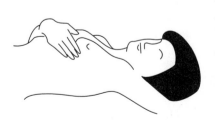

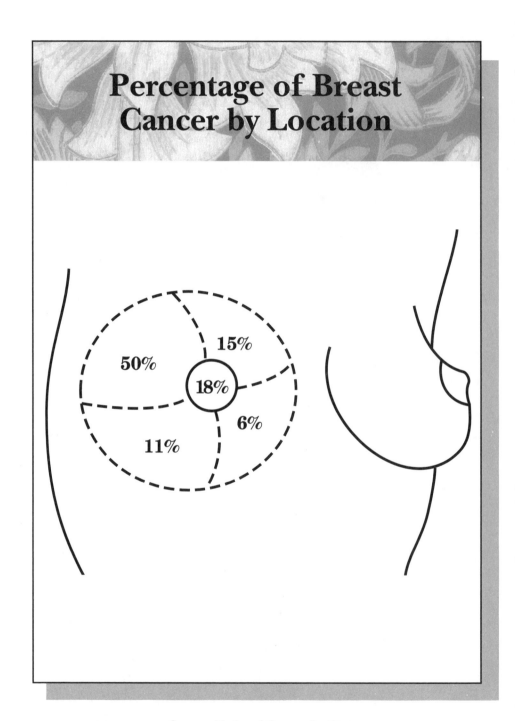

Source: National Cancer Institute

for mammograms and calibrated at least once a year.

- Ask your gynecologist, referring physician, or association if the radiologist has a reliable reputation and is reading at least fifteen mammograms a day.
- Don't have any deodorant, perfume, ointments, or powder on your breasts or underarm area the day of the exam because these substances can distort the picture.
- If you have breast tenderness as a regular part of your menstrual cycle, don't schedule your test within ten days prior to your period. This will avoid discomfort during the compression that the exam requires. If on HRT, wait at least one week after your progesterone replacement before having a mammogram.
- Don't ever have copies of your mammogram films sent for consultation to your physician, gynecologist, or breast specialist. Copies lose a great deal of important definition. Insist on the originals.

NEW IMAGING METHODS

New imaging techniques are improving more and more every day. Some of the most promising include magnetic resonance imaging (MRI), a test that helps to differentiate normal from cancerous tissues by comparing their densities and blood flows. Digital mammography is a process that creates, stores, and enhances mammograms. Scintimammography involves injecting a radioactive tracer which illuminates cancerous tissues using mammographic techniques.

Imaging technology is also being developed for defensive purposes to help find breast cancer in its youngest phases.

At the early stage of trials for effectiveness, you may be able to find Computerized Enhanced Imaging Mammograms and MRIs for breast cancer detection. The BBE — breast bio-physical exam — is on the horizon for non-invasive electrical measurement for breast biopsy and could also be the method of the future for cancer screening.

NEW COMPLEMENTARY SCREENING PROCEDURE

Although saying "Breast Alert™ Differential Temperature Sensor" (BreastAlert) is a mouthful, you need to know about it. BreastAlert is a new complementary screening device that measures the temperature differences between the breasts in order to help detect early signs of potential breast disease. It's safe, comfortable, painless, and takes only fifteen minutes in your health provider's office. The heat differences are immediately available.

Some tumors produce excessive heat. In many cases, this heat may be detectable at the surface of the breast. When used in conjunction with other screening procedures, a difference in temperature of 2 degrees or more between mirror-image regions of the breasts indicates further evaluation may be necessary. Since some tumors can double in size in as short a time as eighty days, having an early and accurate way to measure heat differences in the breasts is useful. Mammograms often aren't able to accurately image through dense breast tissue — particularly for those under fifty — and for those for whom a mammogram is not recommended. Check with your physician for the availability of BreastAlert.

New Diagnostics

Before a mammogram would reveal a cancer problem, a blood/body protein known as p65 can be tested for. When breast cancers are in their very early or formative stages, p65 appears in blood and tissue samples. As of this writing, the clinical trials are not complete, and the test is not universally available. But look for it.

Bracai and bracaii genes have been identified in the last few years and appear to account for 90 percent of the inherited cases—which make up only 1 percent of all breast cancers.

While surgical biopsy is an acceptable procedure to diagnose cancer, several methods that cost less and are less invasive to the body have recently become available. Steriotactic biopsy uses modern imaging techniques to guide a needle moving at extremely high speeds in a biopsy of a suspicious area. Though the pinpointed area may not yet contain a palpable lump, this form of biopsy is accurate, minimally painful, and leaves no scar.

Fine-needle aspiration uses a small, hollow needle to remove cells from an abnormal lump. This process helps to identify and tell the difference between a possibly malignant lesion and a benign (non-cancerous) cyst. A larger needle is used in core biopsy, and a small section of the breast containing the lump is removed.

Recent Breast Cancer Treatment Therapies

New breast cancer treatments are also surfacing. Chemotherapies, for example, can be enhanced by altering the order of various drug administrations and by coordinating the times of treatments with recent surgery or radiation therapy. Bone marrow transplants, as well as Taxol®, a new drug derived from the yew tree, are giving new possibilities and hope for treatment of breast cancer. As for relapse prevention, it has been documented that breast cancer recurrence can be reduced by 50 percent by using a hormonal agent called tamoxifan.

Breast cancer studies continue to confirm lumpectomies with post-surgical radiation and chemotherapy treatments are as effective as radical or modified-radical mastectomies. Early detection, better surgical techniques, radiation, new post-surgery hormonal therapies and less toxic chemotherapy improve survival rates every year.

In some very limited trials, estriol — the weakest form of estrogen — has been reported to arrest breast cancer cells or cause remission.

Support groups, healing circles, prayer, counseling, retreats, seminars, loving friends and family — all are powerful elements to add to any treatment choices.

Keep in mind that the average woman has about a 10 percent risk of developing breast cancer by age eighty and the majority of that risk occurs in the decades after menopause. Don't allow the emotional fears about breast cancer overshadow your attention to preventing or diagnosing lung cancer, colon cancer, heart disease, osteoporosis, or any other less publicized health concerns.

The most up-to-date information on breast cancer is available by telephone at the toll-free numbers listed in Resources.

OSTEOPOROSIS

❧

One of the biggest fears women have about growing older is the prospect of suffering from osteoporosis. And for good reason. The fractures that result from this bone-weakening disease can result in a significant reduction in life quality and lead to debilitation or even death. This is a subject to take seriously, particularly because it develops silently, over a long period of time, without symptoms. Again, early prevention is the key.

IMPORTANT FACTS ABOUT OSTEOPOROSIS

About 300,000 women a year have fractures that cause them to lose their independence for good. It is documented that 51 percent of those who are fifty-five to seventy-four will suffer from some degree of osteoporosis. For women over seventy-five, the number increases to around 75 percent. These statistics should make it clear why you need to know about osteoporosis.

DEVELOPMENT OF OSTEOPOROSIS

Your bones are living structures in need of food and nutrition. They go through a continuous state of what's called "bone remodeling." Certain cells constantly take away the old bone material and other cells repair and rebuild, laying down new bone. Bones deteriorate when new growth is not fast enough to replace the loss of old bone material. The balance is lost between the two steps. The removal of the old, damaged bone stays the same, but the laying down of new replacement bone slows. At menopause, when the estrogen supply decreases, women have to take an active role in preserving their bones. With osteoporosis, new bone is still laid down and it's as strong as younger bone. There's just not enough of it.

BONE LOSS INFORMATION

Most bone loss tends to take place in the first three to eight years of menopause. A woman's natural pre-menopause estrogen supply seems to play a substantial role keeping bones strong. It helps the body absorb calcium, the vital bone-feeding mineral. If the body isn't getting the calcium it needs from diet or supplements, it starts borrowing from the calcium "bank" in your bones. More than 95 percent of your body's calcium is stored there. At the time this occurs, your bones become less dense. They become porous and may actually collapse. When this happens, you can get shorter. When bones go through this change, they become more fragile and fracture more easily.

Osteoporosis can affect us all. This debilitating disease strikes men and women of all ages. There is no immunity.

Prevention is the goal. Prevention is much better than relying on treatment. Before menopause, overly-strenuous exercise, poor nutrition, rapid weight loss, removal of ovaries, pituitary tumors, and anything else that causes estrogen reduction in your system can reduce or stop the normal flow of your periods and can cause rapid bone deterioration. The natural drop in estrogen at menopause will do the same thing. At first no one can see it or feel it. It's only in the later stages that you'll notice the symptoms of gradual loss in height, the "dowager hump," chronic back pain, breathing difficulties, and the lower abdomen thrusting forward.

Around age thirty-five, your bones begin to gradually lose their strength and density at the rate of about 1 percent a year. At menopause and after, between the ages of fifty and sixty, without estrogen replacement and other preventive regimens, such as calcium supplements and weight-bearing exercise, there is a more rapid loss of bone mass. After age sixty, the rate goes down ½ to 1 percent a year. The best way to take good bone-care of yourself is to start supplements and a calcium-rich diet early—many experts say from puberty on. But don't worry. Any time, any age, is a good time to repair and rebuild bone. Once you have this information, you know what can be done. Just be sure to tell your teenage daughters and friends. Spread the word.

WOMEN AT HIGHER RISK

Osteoporosis tends to run in families. But that doesn't mean if your mother or grandmother had it, you will too, or that if your mother or grandmother didn't have it, you won't.

Women with higher risk of osteoporosis are:
- thin;
- blonde;
- of Northern European or Asian origin;
- non-exercising;

- menopausal around forty;
- those with diets low in calcium;
- smokers;
- heavy alcohol drinkers (alcohol is toxic to bones, as well as a contributor to bone loss);
- heavy consumers of cola drinks, fatty foods, processed foods, high meat diets, carbonated beverages, and salty foods — all these increase the loss of calcium when you urinate; and/or
- women who take long courses of cortisone-like drug therapy for asthma, arthritis, or cancer, who may find that calcium has been leached from their bones (the same thing happens to women on excessive doses of thyroid medication or those who have an over-active thyroid).

Remember, however, that only two-thirds of the women who get osteoporosis don't have high-risk profiles.

Girls from puberty onward need to know about calcium and good bone building. Most of our lives we tend to take our bones for granted. Midlife and beyond is payback time. Your bones need you to care for them.

PREVENTING OSTEOPOROSIS

You are well advised to know the types of calcium available and the ways you prefer to take it for your health and comfort considerations.

The National Institutes of Health tell us that most women in America only get about 500 mgs of calcium a day from their diet. This is not enough to build bones or even

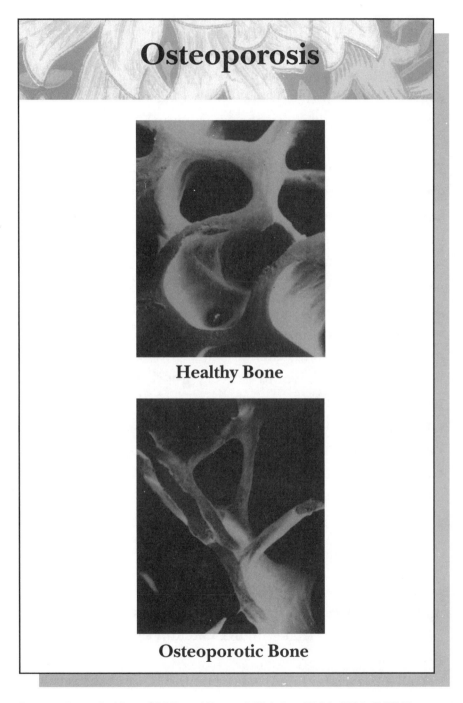

Osteoporosis

Healthy Bone

Osteoporotic Bone

Source: *Journal of Bone & Mineral Research.* Vol. I, p.15-21, 1986, D.W. Dempster.

maintain them. Supplementing calcium is your insurance policy against bone loss. Bone mass is in place by the time you're twenty-three, and most of your body's calcium is stored in your bones. Before menopause, your estrogen supply helps the body to absorb calcium.

Some of the best calcium-rich foods are nonfat milk and yogurt; sesame seeds; sea vegetables such as kelp; leafy greens such as collard, kale, mustard, and turnips; broccoli; and soybean products. Also refer to the calcium food chart in the back of the book.

Leading nutritionists say that after menopause we need to ingest 1000 mgs of calcium daily if on estrogen replacement therapy and 1500 mgs daily without ERT. Most women will need "elemental" or "actual" (these terms mean the same thing) calcium supplements to reach these levels. However, it would be very good for your overall health and disease prevention to try to choose an abundance of calcium-rich foods for your nutritional regimen. Eat small quantities of animal protein, since it can leach calcium from your system. If you like, you can adjust your supplements based on your calcium food intake.

CALCIUM SUPPLEMENTS

Finding calcium sources appropriate for your system and preferences can be confusing. Types of calcium and other ingredients that enhance calcium's effects are mentioned below.

Calcium citrate. Reports say that the body absorbs calcium citrate most easily. Each capsule or tablet contains one-quarter of the elemental calcium a midlife woman needs. It is more digestible than other sources; it's also more expensive. And to get the amount you need usually meant taking frequent doses — usually two capsules three times a day. Caution: Calcium citrate (as well as citrus fruits, drinks, and other citrus products) should not be ingested if you are taking antacids with high aluminum content such as Mylanta®, Maalox®, Amphojel®, AlternaGel®, or Basaljel®. The citrates bind with the antacid's aluminum content to form a new aluminum compound that the intestinal tract easily absorbs and dumps into the bloodstream. This can create a serious health problem in addition to thwarting your attempts to put calcium into your system.

Calcium carbonate. At 40 percent content, it has the highest degree of elemental calcium, but it is not absorbed as well as the citrates and some of the calcium combinations. In addition, carbonates can cause digestive problems, resulting in burping and constipation. Most brands are made from limestone and are lead-free, but others are made from oyster shell which can contain lead if not purified. This can be a problem if you take it for long periods. Calcium carbonate is one of the least expensive to purchase and is the most common calcium supplement available. Although it is a good calcium source, it is not necessarily as effective as some other choices.

Calcium combinations. Some women like to choose supplements that include various kinds of preferred calcium. In these supplements, various calciums are mixed with other ingredients such as vitamin D, magnesium, boron, boric acid, malic acid, manganese, and/or zinc in a highly absorbable amino acid chelate form, sometimes coupled with MCHC (microcrystalline hydroxyapatite). There are experts who feel this is the best possible choice. This kind of supplement (e.g. Osteoform®) can be purchased from your doctor or nutritionist.

Chewable calcium-added antacids. The choices you'll find that don't have aluminum in them are Tums® and Rolaids®. Their calcium source is limestone, and their advantage is that they are an inexpensive, convenient way to get this essential mineral.

Dolomite and bone meal. These so-called natural sources of calcium can be harmful unless they are purified. They may contain amounts of lead, arsenic, cadmium, or mercury that are unsafe in the body when accumulated over time. You won't, however, find this warning information on their labels.

SOME GOOD TIPS FOR TAKING
CALCIUM SUPPLEMENTS

Taking calcium in capsules is the best and most efficient choice for delivering calcium to your body. Other forms are available, and if you do not like to swallow pills, Cal-Mag® is a liquid alternative. But whether you take capsules, tablets, chewables, or liquid, it is recommended that you divide the daily regimen in thirds. Take it throughout the day so you don't overwhelm your calcium absorption system. Also, always take your supplements with food because studies show the results are more effective than taking calcium on an empty stomach.

Whatever form you're taking, it's good to drink a glass

Calcium Recommendations for Women

Age	Dose (mgs)
11 – 24	1,200-1,500
25 – 49	1,000
25 – 49 pregnant, lactating	1,200-1,500
50 – 60 with ERT*	1,000
50 – 60 without ERT*	1,500
65 and older	1,500

*Estrogen Replacement Therapy

Source: National Osteoporosis Foundation, Washington, D.C.

of water at the same time you take your calcium to help move it through the system. Drinking water when you take calcium supplements is also kinder to the kidneys. Six to eight glasses of water a day is good health practice anyway.

During sleep you actually lose calcium. So it's recommended to take about one-third of your last daily dose with some food just before going to bed. It may also soothe your sleep.

Caution: If you have a history of kidney stones or kidney disease, speak to your physician before beginning a calcium regimen. You can probably still take 1,500 mgs of calcium with increased fluid intake, but it would not be recommended for you to ingest more.

Also, if you have food allergies or diabetes, check the labels to see if the supplement contains glucose (sugar), starch (lactose), flavorings, etc. These additives could be harmful.

You'll find most calcium supplements at your local pharmacy, supermarket, or health food store. Special products can be ordered through chiropractors, nutrition specialists, and health advisors.

OSTEOPOROSIS SCREENING TESTS

Many women don't find out they have osteoporosis until they suffer a crippling fracture in their post-menopausal years. Bone density tests can offer revealing information, whether you are in menopause, past menopause, or at risk, regardless of age. For those women at risk who are not taking hormone replacement, bone-building medications, or calcium supplements and who are not engaging in weight-bearing exercise, it's even more important to have a bone density test to determine your current status.

Select the DEXA (Dual-Energy X-Ray Absorptiometry), also known as the QDR (Quantitative Digital Radiography) screening test. This technology is the newest bone density diagnostic tool, and, in Dr. Arpels' expert opinion, "is the screening method of choice." After scanning the body for about twenty minutes, a radiologist can tell whether there is bone loss, where it is, and how severe. It is a painless procedure.

If you have no indications of osteoporosis, you can get a yearly measurement of your urine calcium excretion. This test tells how much calcium your bones are losing. It is not expensive and can give good information. If the urine test yields abnormal results, you would repeat the DEXA/QDR every one to three years and take your annual calcium excretion tests in between.

BUILDING BONE MASS/PREVENTING LOSS

Weight-bearing exercise. Walk. Skip. Jog. Jump rope. Dance. Climb stairs. Use free weights. Use machines if they are available. The kind of exercise that strengthens bones requires your bones to bear the weight of your own bone mass through physical activity or with the resistance of added weights. The idea is to stimulate bone formation by working your muscles against gravity. This involves using weights, dumbbells, weight-resistant pulleys, etc. Even though exercise can cause only a 10 percent increase in bone mass, this can be enough improvement to prevent debilitating fractures. The earlier in your life you start to exercise, the better. But it's never too late to start. Scientific studies have shown that even women in their eighties can build back some bone with the right weight-bearing exercise. So never say "Never."

A cautionary note: If you already have osteoporosis, you should only enter into an exercise program after getting advice from an expert on the subject.

Chiropractic treatments. A knowledgeable, reputable practitioner who has special knowledge about women's midlife and senior health can help with some of the postural problems and joint flexibility. These treatments, however, won't stop bone loss.

Hormone Replacement Therapy. For those women who choose it, HRT has been proven effective for stopping bone loss while increasing bone replacement. Studies show that post-menopausal women who take estrogen for six years or more reduce their lifetime probability of certain types of fractures by 40 percent. Some medical doctors, in fact, strongly urge women who are at risk for osteoporosis to consider HRT, and some include the option of taking small doses of testosterone. The chapter on "Hormone Replacement and Other Options" explains more about this male sex hormone that is also produced by a woman's ovaries and adrenal glands.

The longer you take HRT, the larger the benefit. Dr. Morris Notelovitz, founder of the National Menopause Society, has been successful using a low 0.5 mg dose of Estrace® daily to increase calcium absorption. However, since 4 to 5 percent of the patients on hormone replacement will still have some bone loss, a yearly urine screening is advisable. If the hormone therapy is stopped in five or ten years, however, studies show that bone loss can begin again and the protection against fractures will be decreased. Chapter Two has a full discussion of the benefits and risks of hormone replacement therapy.

Non-hormonal medications. Bisphosphonates have tested very well as bone replacement drugs that also stop the bone-loss phase of osteoporosis. The newly FDA-approved bisphosphonate is known as Alendronate. It is available from Merck as Fosamax® and offers the best choice yet for non-hormonal treatment of osteoporosis. However, look for newer, more user-friendly bisphosphonates that are close to FDA approval.

Bisphosphonates increase bone density while decreasing the incidence of vertebral and hip fractures by 40 to 50 percent. It is required that you take Fosamax orally with eight ounces of water only, on an empty stomach, and not to eat, drink, or lie down for thirty minutes afterward to avoid unpleasant digestive problems and to enhance the effectiveness of the drug. Calcium supplements should not be used along with this medication as they can impair the results. If you have ulcers, gastric difficulties, or problems with your kidneys, this may not be the drug of choice for you. Otherwise, Fosamax is fairly free of side effects.

SERMs stands for Selective Estrogen Receptor Modulators, a relatively recent group of drugs that function somewhat like estrogen in protecting bones from osteoporosis and the heart from cardiovascular disease. They target these body functions without building up the lining of the uterus or causing estrogen-dependent breast cancer tumors to grow more rapidly. Evista®, the brand name for raloxifene, the SERM from Eli Lilly, is now available by prescription. Even though very few side effects have been reported in the study groups, hot flashes appear to occur for some. It should be noted, however, that none of the SERMS undergoing testing at the moment appear to positively enhance mental functioning or the relaxation of blood vessels or have the anti-oxidant effects that estrogen replacement does. There is a good result in bone hip strength with Evista, but the lower spine effect is only 50 percent of that achieved with standard Estrogen Replacement Therapy.

Calcitonin has recently become available as Calcimar®— a nasal spray that is effective, convenient, and affordable. The calcitonin injections of the past, used for the more serious cases of osteoporosis, caused many side effects and were very expensive. This spray, however, is not considered as effective as alendronate for the prevention of fractures.

Combination approach. Some clinical studies have found positive results from a small (.05 mg) dose of micronized estrogen replacement (estradiol) along with a bisphosphonate to achieve the maximum results for the treatment of osteoporosis.

❧

Discuss the choices in this chapter with your health advisor. And remember to look at the "Check-Up Schedule" in the back of this book for more information on tests, foods, and supplements. You'll want to know about these options in order to make the very personal decision about your choices for the prevention or treatment of heart disease, cancer, and osteoporosis.

As I said at the beginning, don't attempt to learn all this the first time — or even the second time — you read the information. A little bit at a time is just fine. Find a pace that's comfortable. Look into other sources. I want to encourage you to help yourself stay well. And hopefully, this timely information will prevent you from becoming seriously ill.

Never forget that an ounce of prevention is worth a pound of cure!

CHAPTER EIGHT

Tackling the Issues— Identity, Habits, and Weight

"Own the heart and soul of who we are."

—*Joan Kenley*

TACKLING THE ISSUES—
IDENTITY, HABITS, AND WEIGHT

WHO ARE YOU?

*W*ho are you? Such a short question — such a big question. One thing today's woman can count on is that the complex answer cannot be carved in stone. Challenges come into our lives from ever increasing directions. The speed of change in the world goes faster and faster. How do we face all this and still define ourselves?

I've never met a woman who isn't searching for something in her life. Something to add: more Being, enhanced worthiness, better education, classier looks, secure identity. Or something to subtract: weight, guilt, shame, bitchiness, inequities, stress. Both lists could go on and on. But when I look at the countless conflicting messages about what society models, requests, and even demands of women today, my heart comes apart at the seams. It's almost impossible not to become overwhelmed if we're consciously — or unconsciously — trying to keep up or keep in step.

Do we ever set aside time in our busy schedules to ponder our deeper natures, desires, and beliefs — the deeply rich colors of who we are? Do we allow grief and sorrow to become our teachers instead of pushing away these gritty emotions until they are safely tucked away somewhere beyond our pain? How many times have we regretted not taking the time to reflect upon the truly delicious moments of our lives? Are we awake enough to savor our living when it's happening?

We could cherish the privilege of growing into wisdom instead of dreading the process of aging. We can accept that our inner beauty, verve, and glow is more powerful than any obsession about external glamour. We must honor the elder women in our families and our communities, allowing them to mentor us into the future. Anne Dosher, Ph.D., the elder to whom I dedicated my "Full Moon Morning" poem (at the end of the first chapter), is a mentor to me and many other women. She has opened my eyes to the spirit of community, the power of the collective, the presence of the elements (fire, air, earth, and water), and the need to honor women's wisdom. Her influence has reminded me that it doesn't matter if our senior women friends are imperfect or don't at times agree with us, it is they who have gone the distance insofar as age is concerned. And in your own aging, you are creating a legacy for those who are following in your footsteps.

It's terrific to have people compliment your looks, voice, talents, brilliance, and style. And you can be remembered wonderfully for those qualities. But when it comes to leaving more profound memories, you can let others become acquainted with your soul's purpose by following your intuition and responding to your inner calling. Seek out your greater self. Stand for who you really are.

Oakland, California, intuition trainer, coach, consultant, and author, Sharon Franquemont (*You Already Know What To Do,* Tarcher/Putnam, to be published in 1999), says:

Intuition is the language of the soul, going beyond normal perception to seize another level of knowing with one glance. This is the glance of your soul. It knows who you are — your search for truth, your encounters with pain, your mastery, and your pure beauty — therefore, it knows what is needed for wisdom and wellness. While the non-linear feminine nature and the soul itself have been associated with inner wisdom, too often healthcare has been identified exclusively with the linear masculine style and the material outer world. Because of this, medical practices in our Western culture have been primarily defined by scientific models. With a very few exceptions, the soul has not been perceived as integral to the healing process and, therefore, not invited into it.

I urge you to change all that. At a minimum invite your soul to be part of your healing team. Intuition can help you accomplish that in two ways:

The first is to tap into the advice of your inner, intuitive healer. We all have an inner healer who knows every nook and cranny of our struggles. Go deep within yourself and ask your inner healer for guidance and help. Responses can come immediately as guiding words, quick images, or strong knowledge that you physically experience in your body. Or later, because of your openness, relevant information and/or inspiration can come from a book, a conversation, music, the media, etc. Keep a record of these messages and pay attention to what they reveal. You do not need to exclude traditional care; what you learn is in addition to other healing modalities not a substitute for it. If the advice from your inner healer and your traditional healthcare givers conflicts, pause briefly before doing anything, do your best to integrate the situation, and seek more information. Never forget your soul knows your path and is on your side.

The second way intuition can help you access your soul is simple: become a wisdom seeker in every aspect of your life. It is my belief that wisdom and wellness are deeply wedded.

Women have a special role to play here. As the archetypal holders of wisdom, we must come forward with our gifts in every arena from care of the planet to care of our bodies. In touch with this understanding, you and all of us already know what to do; without it, we flounder around crying, "I don't know what to do" or "So little can be done." When we say these kinds of things, we are really saying, "I've lost touch with my soul and its guiding wisdom." Women committed to wellness will strike such phrases from their vocabulary and seek to fulfill the promise of their illumination in physical health and total wellness.

What Sharon has so powerfully suggested can bring a working awareness to each day that would add immeasurably to our living. Yet knowing the day-after-day pressures that many of us face, it's clear that a commitment like this would have to be a strong one to carve out the life space to embrace such a focus. But, oh, how glorious the rewards!

And what about your commitment to pleasure? It's a very real need. Don't just fantasize about the exultation of a long, hot bath, the extravagance of shopping leisurely, or the deliciousness of a day to yourself. Why not decide to enrapture your partner, wallow in some scrumptious perfume, or enchant yourself with new ways to play?

Although physicians can't write out a prescription for enjoyment, the endorphins released in the brain during pleasure are essential for optimal wellness. If you had a Self-Delight-O-Meter which measured the amount of daily pleasure you experience on a scale from zero to ten, what would your score be? If your number is low, try to discover why. A reminder — no one should have to give you permission. Search for occasions to have a good belly laugh. Do things on a lark. Find out what enthralls you.

As part of the identity subject, do you ever wonder, "But how do people see me?" Or, "What if my 'radiant soul self' isn't seen because of my image?" If you have reached a place in your life where your interest doesn't include this kind of concern, just skip the image parts of this chapter, heed the health messages, and rejoice. If you have some curiosity about this subject, read on. Paula, age thirty-eight and appearing years younger, moans, "Sure, it's wonderful that I look so good for my age, but inside I feel much older — aches, pains and no energy."

Barbara, who is forty-five, has the opposite problem: "My face started to look like a road map of wrinkles in my early thirties, but I feel younger and have more energy than any of my friends."

Everyone has met the seemingly youthful woman who in reality feels or is years older, and the vital woman who is not as old as we might have imagined. However, society tends to put certain women like Paula and Barbara, as well as countless others, in boxes, projecting assumptions and stories based upon absurd generalities onto them.

What image do you want? What image do you have? Should you care? After all, what does thirty-five, forty-five, fifty-five, sixty-five, etc. look like? None of us can say. Heredity, health habits, and emotional and medical histories all come into play as we add more and more birthdays. We can't alter our aging genes yet, although that possibility appears to be on the medical calendar of the future. What we can do is take advantage of the "here and now" to create the conscious authorship for our inner souls and outer appearance among the choices that are viable and available.

EARLY AGING LIFESTYLE FACTORS

The search for extended youth has been going on since the dawn of time, but no one has been able to stop the clock. While our genes play a gigantic role in looks, health, and aging, a negative environment, diet, and lifestyle can promote early aging. Just know that much of what contributes to aging can be changed:

Stress can cause mental and physical haggardness and increase the possibility of major disease. Dr. Robert S. Eliot, an expert on stress and its impact on our lives, feels that "stress may be the greatest single contributor to illness in the industrialized world." Managing your reactions to stress and choosing to shift negative situations into positive challenges is worth considering. The section on stress management in this chapter addresses this in more detail.

Cigarette smoking causes wrinkles, robs your skin of a healthy glow, and can bring on menopause one or two years early. Smoking is deadly for your heart and lungs, and is a cause of other major health concerns. Even if you've been smoking for years, stopping now can greatly enhance the health and quality of your life as well as your life expectancy.

Heavy alcohol consumption also causes wrinkles. It depletes important vitamins, minerals, and enzymes. It can promote bloating and negatively affect healthy bones and your immune system. Brain and liver functions can also be harmed from heavy drinking, and alcohol can increase your risk of major illness. Your behavior can become inappropriate. For some, however, one alcoholic drink per day may help with their reactions to stress. If you do not have an addiction problem, research suggests regular consumption of small amounts of red wine helps to prevent cardiovascular disease. Alcohol in general increases HDL, the good cholesterol, yet beyond moderation it is unwise in every circumstance.

High-fat diets, junk food, and too much sugar can cause weight gain, bad complexion, and significant health problems, especially heart disease. Even if you felt that you got away with this behavior without adverse side effects early in your life, chances are your metabolism won't be able to handle this continued abuse as you get older. Between the ages of forty-five and fifty-five, most metabolisms drop by 15 percent or more. If a diet of this type doesn't begin to add weight, you still are putting yourself at risk for serious disease.

Inactivity can create loss of muscle mass and tone, joint problems, and stiffness of the spine, as well as decreased flexibility that will slow down your body. Without exercise, you may begin to walk, act, and move in ways that imply an age beyond your actual years.

A negative outlook will limit your horizons and can push people away. It often stimulates unhealthy physical and emotional responses that can create lack of energy, depression, crankiness, mean-spiritedness, and diminished capacity for optimal health. It can isolate you and even shorten your life expectancy.

Mind over Matter

The power of our mind is intimately linked with our overall well-being, and focusing on a healthy mind-set is all part of maintaining a youthful you. If attention is paid to nurturing your mental healthiness, you can slow down the aging process while living with verve and positivity.

Adopt a positive attitude because a joyful, optimistic outlook will add youthfulness to anyone. So will the balanced management of life's work, family, relationships, stresses, and challenges. Psychological well-being, a generous heart, humor in the face of adversity, and the quality of spiritual peace can bring heightened attractiveness to anyone.

Don't worry, inasmuch as a worrisome attitude is never health-positive. We all have the choice to work with the reality of our own personal self-image, health habits, weight management, and the options we find individually comfortable. There are cosmetic aids, surgical enhancers, food and exercise for wellness, and weight specialists for those who care to choose them. A healthy body, a clear mind, and a twinkle in the eye can have a deeper impact than fashion and facelifts. Reveal the beauty that shines from within.

Mental exercise such as learning new skills, reading, memorizing, solving puzzles, and playing mind games stimulates the brain in ways that maintain mental agility as aging occurs.

Eat as if Your Life Depended on It

In addition to mental nurturing and caring, it is essential to remember that indeed, you are what you eat. If there are "miracle remedies" for staying healthy and feeling young, great eating habits are near the top of the list to slow down that march of time.

Consume vegetables daily—fresh if possible. If that sounds difficult or if you don't like veggies, please try to fall in love with them any way you can. Vegetables are considered more protective for good health than any other food category. For those over thirty, the digestive tract usually begins to lose the ability to break down and digest the full nutritional value of raw or slightly cooked vegetables. Thus, steaming or cooking them until they are just beyond crunchy but not limp or soggy is the key. The goal is to soften the cellular structure of the vegetables to allow nutrients to become more available to your system. Five portions each day are recommended.

Lettuce salad—the ever-popular lunch for many women—has many pitfalls. Oil dressings transform this midday meal into the largest single source of fat in most women's diets. But even with lowfat dressings, a plate of lettuce has minimal nutritional value and doesn't offer sufficient food energy to get you through the afternoon.

Salads can be balanced nutritionally if they have lowfat ingredients, an abundance of vegetables and, if you wish, small amounts of turkey, fish, chicken, or tofu. However, oil-filled croutons, bacon, hams, salami, cheeses, and sour cream add a dangerous number of calories and saturated fat grams.

Eat fruit every day suited to your individual energy and digestive responses—optimally, five fresh servings. Cook them if digesting them raw causes bloating or indigestion. The health protective value isn't lost by cooking, although people used to think so.

If you have blood sugar ups and downs plus energy crashes after a fruit snack, eat your fruits, fresh or cooked, combined with a complex carbohydrate such as multigrain bread and a small amount of protein for a sustained energy snack. Some nutritionists recommend eating fruit after meals for best assimilation. If you still have energy fluctuations, you may have to limit fruit intake to two or three portions a week or find the frequency that suits you best. Drinking fruit juices can influence a rise and fall in energy even more than whole fruits. But if you have a preference for fruit juice, you may want to experiment with a glass of one-third juice and two-thirds water to see how your energy is affected. Trying these easy suggestions may smooth out your energy problems.

If you don't have energetic or digestive problems with fruit, eat four or five daily servings. It's best to eat fresh fruits and adjust the type of fruits as availability and seasons change. If you are choosing packaged, canned, or frozen fruits, check labels to detect sugar content. Sugar can add unwanted calories and reactions.

If you have trouble controlling your energy ups and downs or have problems with weight loss, you may need to watch the type of carbohydrates you ingest. Study the following charts and try to avoid or minimize your intake of fruits and vegetables with high carbohydrate content (15 to 20 percent). Instead, focus on eating more of those fruits and vegetables that are only 5 or 10 percent carbohydrates.

Whole grain/unrefined breads, cereals, pasta, rice and other grains, potatoes, and beans should be included based on your level of carbohydrate sensitivity. Do carbohydrates make you feel bloated, sleepy, or cause you to be hungrier than usual? If so, you may want to eat more vegetables and protein while reducing the amount of these foods. A slice of bread or a fistful of rice can be a satisfactory serving when you're eating a healthy variety of foods.

Limit your refined sugar intake. Linda Prout, nutritional consultant, offers an excellent summary about the effects of sugar consumption:

It is estimated that one third of the population is sugar sensitive. If you are among that one out of three, you will feel its effects. That may mean irritability, fatigue, depression, confusion, memory loss.

I used to say the single most important thing most people can do to improve their diet is cut down on fats. I now

Carbohydrate Sensitivity Guide to Fruits and Vegetables

Eat Heartily—5%*

Fruits

avocados	honeydew	cantaloupe
strawberries	watermelon	

Vegetables

asparagus	eggplant	pumpkin
bean sprouts	endive	radishes
beet greens	kohlrabi	spinach
broccoli	lettuce	string beans
cabbages	mustard greens	summer squash
cauliflower	okra	tomatoes
celery	olives	(ripe) turnips
cucumbers	peppers	watercress

Eat Reasonably—10%*

Fruits

blackberries	peaches	grapefruits
oranges	tangerines	

Vegetables

beets	olives (green)	brussel sprouts
onions	carrots	rutabaga
leeks	winter squash	

*Carbohydrate percentage

Source: *Human Nutrition Service and Agriculture Handbook.* U.S. Department of Agriculture. Adapted by Emily K. Wolman.

Carbohydrate Sensitivity Guide to Fruits and Vegetables

Eat Sparingly—15%*

Fruits

apples	mulberries	apricots
pears	blueberries	pineapples
cherries (sour)	plums	grapes
raspberries	loganberries	

Vegetables

artichokes	parsnips	peas

Avoid—20%

Fruits

bananas	cherries (sweet)	figs (fresh)
grape juice	prunes (fresh)	

Vegetables

corn	hominy	kidney beans
lima beans	navy beans	potatoes

*Carbohydrate percentage

Source: *Human Nutrition Service and Agriculture Handbook.* U.S. Department of Agriculture. Adapted by Emily K. Wolman.

193

say it may be sugar causing you more health problems than the fat. Watch your intake of refined sugars: sucrose, fructose, corn sweeteners, invert sugar and the foods most often made with them: cookies, candy, cake, frozen yogurt, etc.

Refined sugars deplete the body's stores of B vitamins, magnesium and chromium — the brain/mind/energy nutrients. A high sugar intake is linked with a variety of mental complaints, from depression and fatigue to violent behavior. Over-eating sugar is also linked with diabetes, low blood sugar, reduced immunity, obesity, bowel disease, colon cancer and heart disease. Sugar not only may lead to physical disease and weight gain but adverse mind and mood changes.

Perhaps just as disconcerting, sugar may accelerate the aging process. Studies show refined sugars reduce the lifespan of animals. Sweets are thought to increase oxidation — the aging process implicated with heart disease and cancer. Refined sugars include sucrose (white table sugar), brown sugar, fructose, corn syrup, and high fructose. They are often added to cereals, cookies, muffins, cakes, pies, juices and sauces.

If you're not carbohydrate sensitive, Linda suggests that you snack on crackers, baked chips, popcorn, whole grain breads, soups, vegetables, and fruits. Those who have reactions to certain carbs should combine small portions of protein and olive oil with vegetables and fruits for snacking, limiting or avoiding the ones mentioned in the preceding charts.

Fiber in the diet can improve blood sugar levels, reduce blood levels of fat and cholesterol, and lower risk of colon cancer. The daily consumption of dietary fiber should be 20 to 50 grams.

Oil that is unsaturated is needed in small amounts in your diet. Lowfat eating does not mean no-fat eating. Olive, canola, grape, and walnut oils are excellent for you. Also use the important essential fatty acids (EFAs) found in wheat germ or fish oils, as well as in vitamin E or primrose oil capsules. The EFA oils need to be purchased when they are fresh, and they must be refrigerated or they will become rancid. You'll find all essential fatty acids — in capsules or bottles — at your health food store, drugstore, or grocery store.

Protein sources come in varying types worthy of consideration. It is suggested that you limit your red meat intake to a few times a month. Fish, poultry, and tofu can be eaten frequently, and eggs are good a few times a week if you are not on a very restricted regimen that excludes them. Many healthy people are consuming 3 to 4 oz. portions of protein at each meal for daily health and energy. When you fuel your body with good nutrition, you function better and don't feel deprived.

Tofu is an important protein staple to consider, particularly for vegetarians. It's made from soybean curd and is becoming more and more popular as people are trying to consume less meat. Three main types of tofu are available in most food stores:

- *Firm tofu* is solid, dense, and one most commonly used as a meat substitute. It's perfect for burgers, sausages, "meatloaf," hearty soups, stir-frying, and grilling — wherever you want it to hold its shape. Of the three types, firm tofu is highest in protein, fat, and calcium.
- *Soft tofu* works well in recipes that call for blending and in soups, sauces, and dressings. Lower in fat and thus not as solid as firm tofu, this form allows for much creativity in the kitchen.
- *Silken tofu* is perfect for pureed products with finer textures such as ice creams, yogurts, and custards.

Nutrients Found in 4 Ounces of Tofu

	Firm Tofu	Soft Tofu	Silken Tofu
Calories	120	86	72
Protein (grams)	13	9	9.6
Carbohydrates (grams)	3	2	3.2
Fat (grams)	6	5	3.4
Saturated Fat (grams)	1	1	—
Cholesterol	0	0	0
Sodium (milligrams)	9	8	76
Fiber (grams)	1	—	—
Calcium (milligrams)	120	130	40
Iron (milligrams)	8	7	1
% of calories from protein	43	39	53
% of calories from carbohydrates	10	9	17
% of calories from fat	45	52	30

Source: Composition of Foods: Legumes and Legume Products.
Human Nutrition Service and Agriculture Handbook.
U.S. Department. of Agriculture. Adapted by Emily K. Wolman.

All forms of tofu are rich in protein, low in saturated fat, and contain no cholesterol. High in B vitamins and iron, tofu can also be a good source of calcium if a calcium salt is used in the curdling process. Tofu is low in sodium, and, for some women, it can help to reduce hot flashes. Though measurements differ between the three forms, the basic rule is the softer the tofu, the lower the fat content. Review the chart on the next page for an easy glance at the terrific nutritional benefits you can receive from various types of tofu.

Dairy products are good calcium sources. Servings of lowfat and nonfat milk, cheese, and yogurt are recommended daily if you aren't on a dairy-free regimen. If so, choose soy, or rice "milk" products.

DIGESTIVE CONCERNS

As we age, there are other food considerations to keep in mind. For example, hydrochloric acid, normally available in our stomachs for efficient digestion, decreases as time goes by. Explore with a nutritionist if any HCL supplements, available at pharmacies and health stores, would be helpful. If you have heartburn, explore standard or alternative anti-acid remedies. Note that some ulcers are now linked to bacteria and can be cured with antibiotics. Over time, changes in your digestive tract may also cause more gas in your intestines. Try commercially-sold Beano®, a food enzyme dietary supplement, or other such products that reduce flatulence and gaseous intestinal reactions. It is often preferable to consider lunch as your major meal with a light supper during the evening to maintain health and proper weight.

Think of the food you eat the same way you would think of a drug you take. For instance, if you are using something for a headache every three hours to manage the pain, you relate one action to the other result. Food fuels your energy, mental sharpness, and healthy functioning in much the same time-oriented way.

In other words, try to balance the intake of the foods you need. If you fill your protein, carbohydrate, and fat requirements at breakfast, that will have no effect on your afternoon nutritional needs. If you have little or nothing at lunch or overload on calories, your fuel supply goes out of balance, and you begin robbing or shutting down your energy bank account. Count on each meal to affect your body for two to five hours, depending on your needs and what you choose to eat. One of the health advantages of the way many French people eat is that they normally include choices from all food groups at each meal.

EXERCISE ENCOURAGEMENT

Physical exercise is your magic health-bullet. It strengthens your heart. You breathe better. Your circulation is stronger. Your eyes, face, and skin look more vital. Your muscles become toned. You carry yourself more confidently. So, you think you hate exercise? Hate is often like fear. Once you put that hate to some reality tests, it may not seem so awful. When you truly investigate what type of exercise could appeal to you, trying the path of least resistance at first may actually encourage other choices later.

During midlife, when estrogen levels go down, muscle strength often decreases. Conscious focus on muscle toning becomes very important to maintain your strength and vitality. Exercise helps to guard against aches and stiffness. It's vital for preventing serious health problems including osteoporosis, heart disease, and obesity. In the long run, regular exercise can help women keep their independence well into their golden years. Some experts say that older women who exercise regularly may have bodies that are as much as twenty years younger than women who don't.

It's always best to start with something simple, like walking around your neighborhood or on a treadmill. What you need to do most is just start moving. Even getting on your feet more often each day would help. Three or four days a week, walk somewhere. To the store, between stores, to a friend's house, or five extra blocks to a sandwich shop near work. Some women use their moving time as a way to socialize. Have "Power Walks" with friends or colleagues instead of "Power Lunches."

Cheryl Pombo-Soda, who owned an outstanding fitness center in Oakland for fifteen years, is now an American College of Sports Medicine Certified Personal Fitness Trainer specializing in working with women over forty. She tells us that "more important than what you do is the regularity with which you do it. There's nothing wrong with starting any program — of which your health advisor approves — at your own individual pace. Maybe five minutes three times a week, moving up to ten minutes, then twenty."

But if exercise is so great, why is it so hard to do? Why did 64 percent of those polled in a recent survey say they wanted to exercise but couldn't find the time? Cheryl explains:

One reason is that we often want instant fitness and are not willing to invest the time to do the job right. The most important thing when you're starting a regular exercise program is to give yourself time to develop results. You don't need to follow everyone on your block to aerobics class. Such classes might not provide the right exercises for you. Most importantly, you must schedule exercise into your weekly calendar of activities to develop a routine. Then commit yourself to finding some joy in it — in addition to the great health results.

As we grow older, not only does our metabolism lose efficiency each year, but our daily activity level often becomes less physical and more sedentary. If you find that you have gained extra pounds and want to plan a weight loss program, you will want to choose an exercises that works for your size, abilities, and physical condition. This regimen needs to be planned carefully and purposefully. As soon as you start feeling the benefits of exercise, you may find it hard to give it up. The most successful weight programs combine exercise with sensible eating. Remember that losing "only" a pound a week can result in a fifty-pound weight loss in a year.

Movement to get your heartbeat and metabolism activated is one part of the picture. Weight-bearing exercises for muscle and bone strength are just as important as getting your heart pumping regularly. Any exercise is better than no exercise. And don't be caught off guard by charts that indicate how much activity burns off how many calories and conclude that it's just not worth the effort. The overall combination of the right kind of food management and your individualized plan, along with the support of a friend, doctor, or health advisor can make a great combination for success.

Also, don't be fooled by the calorie information on electronic exercise equipment, which may be giving you inaccurate figures, depending on how the machine is calibrated. Personal trainer and professional dancer Diane McKallip says that, "many treadmills, stairclimbers, and stationary bicycles have a readout at the end of the session about calories burned. At best, these numbers are a very rough approximation of energy expenditure. Many factors contribute to an individual's workout results, such as your metabolic rate, level of fitness, and how much muscle mass you have."

SKIN REMEDIES

Skin is a living, breathing organ, the largest organ in our bodies. But we tend to take it for granted. Then one day we wake up and are surprised to see the wrinkles. Much of your skin's condition is genetic, but much is also under your control. Some women spend a good part of their lives harming their skin with sun, harsh soaps, and chemicals. The skin can also be robbed of its vitality with alcohol, caffeine, carbonated soft drinks, and poor diet. What's more, skin naturally loses plumpness over the years. Wrinkles result. Estrogen depletion also plays a role. As your estrogen levels become lower, the elasticity of your skin's connective tissue is reduced, causing sags and wrinkles. Estrogen replacement therapy, hormone creams, the new skin care products, and aloe or vitamin E moisturizers can help skin feel soft and look moist and smooth. You can't stop the years, but there are things you can do to improve your skin's vitality.

Drink lots of water because it is truly the single greatest help for your skin and your health. Most experts suggest six to eight glasses a day. Water helps your system in many ways, and one of them is to feed your skin the nutrients it needs. Water also aids in eliminating toxins and waste products from your system while contributing to the healthy functioning of your vital organs. Since you don't want to flood your system with more than it can handle, drink about four ounces every half hour and only sip water with meals. If you feel that drinking more water makes you feel bloated, stay with it for a few days. Not only will you develop a healthy thirst for water, but in time it should prove to be a useful remedy for eliminating bloating and excess water retention.

ADVICE FROM A SKIN SPECIALIST

Mary Thé, an outstanding aesthetician in the San Francisco Bay Area and owner of the Mary Thé Skin Care Salon, shares her expertise with us:

> *An important point overlooked by most women over forty is that having drier skin does not mean you need to run out and buy a heavier moisturizing cream. Just the opposite is true. You will need a lighter texture and more nourishing products. Heavier creams are useful as protectors when swimming in chlorinated water, engaging in extended outdoor activity, or exposing yourself to cold winter temperatures. These protective creams should be applied on top of your nourishing, lighter moisturizer.*
>
> *Fortunately, new bio-technology and high-tech methods are helping manufacturers develop products and treatments as never before. We have very effective ways to preserve and maintain the appearance and condition of the skin. Regular maintenance is the single most important consideration for midlife women over thirty-five.*
>
> *The available choices for skin care can become confusing without knowledgeable advice. Just because various cosmetic products contain the same active ingredients, they are not necessarily equally beneficial. The quality of the raw materials, processing methods, pH balance, and proportion of active ingredients all contribute to the results you get.*

Mary also advises, "Learn to listen to what your skin is telling you and be flexible to change your routine accordingly. Seek guidance from a professional who will teach you how to take better care of your skin. And be wary of falling too easily for the promotion and hype of some cosmetic manufacturers."

WORST PROBLEM FOR SKIN

Your skin's very worst enemy — in the past, present, and future — is the sun. Those long hours you may have spent tanning on the beach or in the tanning booth can make you wrinkle sooner. Solar rays also make your skin loose, leathery, and splotchy. And they can cause skin cancer.

You can't undo the hours you've already spent sunbathing. But you can choose to greatly reduce this warm weather pastime or even stop it altogether. If you yearn to have a tanned face and body, there are tanning cosmetics that are safe and won't turn your skin orange as did some of the early products. It is not recommended to use tanning salons under any circumstances.

Use sun block everyday. Apply a sunscreen with at least and SPF 15 that blocks both the UVA and UVB rays of the sun. You would be well advised to protect your face and all other exposed body parts, especially your neck, upper chest, forearms, and tops of your hands. Even on a cloudy day, quite a large percentage of the UV rays reach the earth and can damage your skin.

Some tinted moisturizers and makeup bases contain sun-blocking ingredients, but usually not enough. You'll find they're not necessarily calibrated for the broad spectrum of protection you will find in the appropriate sunscreens. If you have sensitive skin, you many want to try a non-chemical sunscreen containing zinc oxide and titanium dioxide. When you're outside, whatever sun protection you're using must be reapplied several times throughout the day, more often if you're perspiring or swimming.

Wear UVA and UVB protection sunglasses. The appropriate sun-protecting glasses can help prevent eye damage and cataracts. If you want to reduce squinting, which causes strain as well as lines around your eyes, wear a big floppy hat to shade your eyes even more.

Extended exposure to sun has the significant danger of causing skin cancer. Basal-cell and squamous-cell carcinomas can be easily and successfully treated when diagnosed early. The rarer and more dangerous melanoma skin cancer is fast-spreading and life-threatening. The frequency of all of these cancers is on the rise. One theory is the diminishing ozone layer and the resulting increase in ultraviolet rays in the atmosphere. One out of six women will probably develop the basal/squamous-cell skin cancer. Those with blonde or red hair, who also burn easily from the sun, have a double risk of skin cancer.

The *San Francisco Chronicle* reported in June 1994 that "self-examination can help to catch dangerous skin cancers before they become serious. J. Ramsey Mellette, M.D., a melanoma specialist at Rose Medical Center in Denver, says that melanomas have a different appearance than normal moles. While normal moles are small, uniform in color, and regularly contoured, melanomas are usually asymmetrical with scalloped borders and variegated color. Basal and squamous cancer may appear as red areas that are scaly and itchy."

PRODUCTS TO REJUVENATE AGING SKIN

For women concerned with aging skin, alpha hydroxy acids and the prescription medication cream Retin-A® have been the products most used. The 1996 release of the new prescription product, Renova®—tretinoin-based like Retin-A, but milder—adds to the choices for reducing fine facial wrinkles, brown spots and surface roughness.

Glycolic, lactic, and other alpha-hydroxy acids (AHAs) are fruit acids that have become the non-prescription rage for youthful skin, but their use should be monitored by a skin professional. They are used in facial peels and other skin preparations to help soften and improve skin tone, and to remove flaking or dry, dead skin cells on the surface. AHAs can promote the growth of new skin cells for a smoother and less wrinkled look. Lactic acid formulas are suggested for those with more sensitive faces. Sometimes the products can be alternated seasonally to meet changing skin needs. AHAs are considered safe during pregnancy.

Retin-A is known for reducing fine wrinkles, clearing up acne, fading age spots, reducing blemishes, restoring collagen formation, and producing rosier skin. For some, this is a fabulous product. For others, it can make the skin too dry, red, and scaly. Doctors who prescribe it should customize the strength and frequency of use for each woman. Some women can't tolerate it no matter what the adjustment is. A Retin-A program needs to be physician-monitored and should not be used by pregnant women. Those planning to have children must stop their regimen four to eight weeks prior to pregnancy.

Renova is a newly available prescription cream that is finding a great deal of satisfied users. It is made from the very same base as Retin-A but has a milder, more moisturizing formula. It appears to be a breakthrough for those whose skin is too sensitive to use Retin-A. Be careful about applying other facial creams immediately before or after Renova. Jonathan Weiss, assistant professor of dermatology at Emory University, says that, "chemically, Renova can become deactivated by any cream not compatible with it." So if you want to use AHAs in combination with Renova, apply the AHA cream in the morning and Renova at night.

If you get rashes and/or blemishes or red-chapped skin from the above products, get professional advice about adjustments or a change of treatment. If you want to refine or customize your Retin-A program, Dr. Juris Bunkis, an esteemed professional in the field of aesthetic and reconstructive surgery in Danville, California, recommends the following technique:

> *Wash your face before retiring in the evening. After your face is dry, a small, pea-sized dab of Retin-A should be spread carefully over the entire face, including eyelids. Then go to bed without adding any other moisturizer or cream. After showering and drying the face in the morning, close inspection will help determine how much Retin-A to apply that evening, based on the color of the face: slight pinkness and pinkness — same amount; redness and excess redness — use less or skip a night; no reaction — add a little more that evening. All users should apply sunblock and choose makeup with sunblock.*

Other products to consider that can nourish the skin and work in conjunction with either AHAs, Retin-A, or Renova treatments are over-the-counter creams and serums. Some are reported to have good results improving facial skin with or without other regimens. Generally speaking, the serums usually contain a higher percentage of active ingredients and can penetrate more easily. They are, therefore, considered the most effective way to nourish the skin.

Collagen injections from a reputable dermatologist or plastic surgeon is another choice for wrinkle reduction. You must be tested beforehand to check for allergies and reactions. Also, injections of your own fat cells can fill in facial wrinkles. But these expensive procedures only give temporary improvement. In fact, some experts feel collagen may not be a good substance to put in your body. Your own fat cells are considered to be safer and can last longer if you have several treatments.

GREAT TIPS FOR LOOKING GOOD

Often a suggestion from someone else's regimen can become another person's great idea. There are new things under the sun, moon, and stars these days. Tried and truisms come around again, maybe with a fresh slant. Women's magazines are timely resources. It's fun to venture into a different approach to viewing — or doing — yourself. If you're having a bad hair day, a bad skin day, a bad food day, or a bad feeling day, it can be mood-lifting to shift your attention to a self-enhancing something that will please you.

SOME SUGGESTIONS FOR LOOKING YOUR BEST:

Excessive showering, bathing or sauna time can rob the skin of natural oils. If that seems to be the case for you, clean your major perspiration areas daily — feet, crotch, groin, underarms, neck, and face — and space your full bathing habits based on your skin's response. If you encounter major overall sweating or grime on a daily basis, showers and bathing can be followed with body oils or moisturizers.

Super-fatted soaps or pH-balanced, low-alkaline ones are easier on the skin than regular soap. For example, Cetaphil®, found in drugstores, is a good non-stripping, non-irritating facial cleanser. Some women prefer a non-soap facial cleansing bar, gel, lotion, or cream.

Applying a moisturizer while your skin is still slightly damp helps seal in moisture. You then have the choice of putting another light moisturizer on top of your makeup, whether you decide to use powder or not.

Temporary "cosmetic skin plumpers" for smoothing facial wrinkles are available at many cosmetic counters. If you're having trouble with lipstick seeping into vertical lip crevices around your mouth, look for lip plumpers and lipstick sealers.

Your licensed aesthetician, cosmetologist, plastic surgeon, or dermatologist has various methods and degrees (light, medium, and deep) of **facial peeling** which can help to eliminate or soften some facial lines and refresh the texture of your skin. Deep chemical peels, normally used for pitted or scarred tissue, should be performed only once in a lifetime to maintain healthy, good-looking skin, and only after careful consultation with a reputable professional. Bleaching creams and chemical / laser techniques are available for removal of brown spots, depending on the location.

Dermatologists and plastic surgeons can remove moles as well as "skin tags" which can start to appear as aging occurs.

Regular facials and skin maintenance techniques are offered by licensed, reputable skin care professionals. These experts can enhance all aspects of any facial beauty regimen. They can also safely dye your eyebrows and lashes.

"Permanent" eyeliner, eyebrow, and lip color can be applied by a permanent make-up professional. These choices can help you feel more "wash and go" if daily makeup is bogging you down and if you can't see as well to make artful and precise applications. However, this pigment usually fades somewhat, especially from the eyelids, and may have to be reapplied every three years or so. Be sure you have reliable recommendations for the person you choose to do these procedures because the field is not licensed.

If **contact lenses** appeal to you, the monovision method (dominant eye gets a distance lens, other eye has the reading correction) or bifocal lenses can help you drop those reading glasses. If you already wear lenses, estrogen foods or estrogen replacement therapy can help your eyes stay moist if menopause has caused them to be too dry for your usual lens comfort, or if you're just beginning to wear them at this time of your life.

Fingernail strength and health can change as you grow older. If your nails are breaking or splitting, Ten-Effex®, Nailtique®, and other such fingernail-strengthening products can make a marked improvement when used alone or as a base and top coat with polish. Natural or colorful polish can also act as nail protectors or to simply beautify nails. But polish colors you've used in the past may not be the best choice as time goes by, if the skin color and texture of your hands has changed.

A non-surgical facial enhancement recommended and used by the Mary Thé Skin Care Salon in San Francisco is the **Micro-current Facial Treatment.** Mary explains it as a "must know" technique that can significantly help facial appearance.

> *The micro-current device I use produces a very low electrical current. These treatments have been used in sports medicine both as a pain reliever and healing method. Celebrities use it as their secret facial revitalizer. The micro-current treatments take the stress away from the facial muscles by re-educating the muscles to normalize themselves. This means that a tense muscle learns to relax and a relaxed muscle learns to wake up, but not become tense. A series of treatments is necessary for long-lasting results. But before a special event, a single session can work wonders.*

PLASTIC SURGERY INFORMATION

Dr. Juris Bunkis' comments come from a broad range of experience in the field of plastic surgery:
1) Cosmetic surgery can be used to enhance one's appearance but great care must be taken to choose

a well-qualified plastic surgeon who not only is board-certified by the American Board of Plastic Surgery, but also specializes in aesthetic surgery.

2) Prospective plastic surgery patients must have proper motivation and realistic expectations. There are no techniques that can make a woman of fifty years look exactly like she did when she was twenty-five. A plastic surgeon can help a person look better by tightening facial and neck skin, reducing facial wrinkles, removing unwanted skin and bags from the eye area, improving a nose or chin, removing unwanted fat deposits or sagging skin, and enlarging or reducing breasts. However, any interested person is advised to take the time to find the appropriate surgeon and to visit the surgeon to discuss the problem before deciding whether surgery is the best solution.

Dr. John E. Emery, a prominent plastic surgeon who owns The Emery Clinic in San Francisco, offers the following descriptions of various procedures:

The forehead lift: A surgical procedure used to lift saggy eyebrows that crowd already tired-looking skin and to remove the stigma of looking cross by eliminating the muscles that create frowning. Scarring on the scalp behind the hairline can sometimes cause see-through scarring if your hair is thin, so be aware that this surgery may limit your hairstyling options. However, some surgeons make their incisions in front of the hairline on the forehead to prevent this limitation.

Implants to the face and chin: A variety of facial implants can give balance to an aging face. They are designed to create more fullness over the cheekbone area, as well as in the mid-face where fat has diminished with age. Implants are also successfully used to improve the chin line which is altered with aging by bony absorption in the jaw. An enhanced jaw line helps to improve the neck, which is itself frequently helped by the removal of fat combined with muscle tightening. Chin reductions can also help to improve a protruding chin.

Nasal enhancement: This procedure is well received because it gives a balance and softness to the face for those who have noses that look too severe.

Lip enhancement: As we age, the relationship between the upper lip and the teeth may change so that the thinner upper lip hangs over the teeth. A pleasing result is achieved by lifting the lip by removing a section of lip skin, either along the vermilion — the red line — or just beneath the nose. The newly positioned lip can be plumped up somewhat by implanting one's own tissue in the lip, a dermo-fat graft, or more recently by the careful implantation of a material called Gortex.

The degree of satisfaction following a surgical procedure will depend largely on how bad the problem was before the surgery, what your expectations were regarding the outcome of the surgical procedure, and whether the surgeon delivered the expected results based on your discussion prior to surgery.

Dr. Emery concludes, "Cosmetic surgery is the 'icing on the cake' that can bring a smile to your face and years of pleasure, providing that all of the ingredients — the patient, the skill of the doctor, the operative planning and an ideal healing response — are there."

A new liposuction technique, the ultrasonic-assisted liposuction (UAL), now permits large-scale removal of fat — up to twenty pounds at once. One of the pioneering plastic surgeons using this new technique, George Commons, M.D., of Palo Alto, tells us that the biggest advantage of UAL is that he uses ultrasonic waves to liquefy fat cells before they are suctioned out. This procedure, therefore, leaves many of the nerves and blood vessels, which are often damaged by traditional liposuction techniques, intact. The UAL method also allows the surgeon to work in areas of the body usually considered difficult to sculpture, such as the waist and upper back. Decisions about whether to have UAL or traditional liposuction must include awareness of the potential discomfort involved and the fact that recovery may take many weeks or months.

Above all, remember this: balance is everything. Only you can know what motivates you — vanity or healthy personal preferences. It's a personal choice whether to have plastic surgery or not. For instance, wrinkles can be trophies, reminders of the years you've lived and of the millions of times you've smiled, scowled, squinted, and scrunched your eyebrows. On the other hand, you can choose to soften or get rid of some wrinkles in order to feel more attractive. You decide.

HAIR CHANGES AND PROBLEMS

Hair changes can occur because of poor health or medical reasons. Most thinning hair comes from just getting older, the hormone changes at menopause and then only for some. And with or without any hair loss on your head, you may find hair appearing in other places you'd rather it wouldn't, like your chin.

Your hair has to eat, just like your body. Estrogen helps feed blood and oxygen to your hair roots. When your estrogen levels drop and stress levels increase, or activities

212

expose you to drying elements, your hair gets hungry. Maybe you aren't feeding your hair well enough with the food you eat. One or two daily tablespoons — or the capsule equivalent — of an essential fatty acid such as flax seed oil can help. These are the type of fats needed for good health and for keeping hair, skin, and soft tissues nice and moist. Taking the mineral supplement silica can help strengthen hair, nails, and skin. If you are at an age when estrogen replacement is part of your regimen choice, estrogen can often contribute to maintaining hair luster.

Your hair may have more than hunger pangs. It may finally be giving in to a lifetime of exposure to sun, wind, rain, swimming pools, and pollutants in the air. A change of shampoo, conditioner, and hairspray may do wonders. Many times, the wrong products have given women the wrong idea about their hair and what can be done with it.

Do something bold. Think about a new way of wearing your hair. Look into hair braiding or the hair weaving, "magic hair fillers." Rogaine® — the registered name for the drug minoxidil — has been a popular product for balding men, and now is recommended for certain women who experience thinning hair.

If you decide to use hair color to make a change or cover gray, remember that some inferior color products are drying. So try the products recommended by a salon or hair colorist or have your hair colored by a professional, if possible. A new, long-overdue female baby boomer product is Hair Mascara®, to touch up the hard-to-color hairline around the forehead and face between colorings. The Christian Dior® product comes in twenty colors (there are other brands as well), and you can also use the wand to streak in interesting highlights.

You'll find many women are choosing to celebrate gray —
also a great choice. Find a way to work with your hair. You'll
be surprised what choices are available once you put your
mind to it. And you'll feel better when your mane pleases
you. There's nothing quite like good hair days!

FACIAL HAIR CONCERNS

Facial hair growth originates from the male hormone
testosterone. All women produce a certain amount of this
hormone, but in much smaller amounts than men. When
estrogen production is lowered because of menopause, a
new "hormone mix" develops. One result can be unwanted growth — sometimes of tough, coarse hair — in places
you least want it — on your face, upper lip, chin, and chest,
for example. Many women tweeze these offending strays.
Other solutions are to bleach, wax, shave, or use hair
removal creams made especially for delicate skin. A reputable licensed electrologist can remove the hairs by killing
the root of each follicle. For some, this can be time-con-
suming, expensive, and sometimes damaging to the skin.
The new needleless, radio-frequency electrolysis treatments
are another choice. Note: unless the hair follicle is des-
troyed completely, the hair will regrow in the same place,
not to mention that there will be a need to remove the new
hair that continues to develop.

DENTAL CARE

Dentistry, specifically cosmetic dentistry, offers excellent options for improving the appearance of your teeth.
Women at menopause and after can find that their gums
and teeth are affected by the decrease in estrogen — loos-
er teeth, more sensitive gums, etc. Dr. Mark McMahon, a

noted specialist in cosmetic dentistry with offices in Los Angeles, tells us about aesthetic/corrective dental procedures as well as hygiene:

Whitening systems: For healthy teeth that have been stained by such daily activities as smoking or drinking coffee, there are a number of treatments available. Aging tends to yellow teeth, and the right color of whiteness for your coloring can add sparkle to your appearance.

Over-the-counter whiteners can be helpful in some cases. However, they are not all the same quality and could cause harm if used improperly. Your dentist can provide a service that is many times more effective than the over-the-counter systems. For maximum safety and more dramatic results, your dentist's "home-supervised" procedures use a custom-made mouth tray and stronger whitening agents.

Bonding: For chips in your teeth or other small defects, a common remedy is known as composite bonding or resin restorations. This is a one-visit procedure which uses light-cured, acrylic materials to precisely match the color of the surrounding teeth. Bonding is an economical solution to simple cosmetic defects such as chips and small spaces, but it can chip or become stained or discolored. For these reasons, bonding may need to be repaired or replaced in three to seven years.

Porcelain veneers: A study conducted at the University of Ontario called porcelain veneers "the most successful restorative technique in the history of the profession." What are they? They are the state-of-the-art in improving and beautifying smiles. A porcelain veneer is a wafer-thin piece of porcelain created to look and act just like real tooth enamel. Completed over two office visits, this technique is a bit more expensive than bonding but last much longer and are more like your own teeth. On the first visit, the teeth are prepared by the dentist and a mold is made of your teeth. The mold is sent to a dental laboratory where the porcelain veneers are finished to match the specifications set by the dentist. When the veneers are ready, the patient returns to the office and they are permanently applied to the teeth.

The cosmetic improvements attainable with porcelain veneers are so dramatic that a person's whole attitude can change as a result of the treatment. A person who is unable or unwilling to smile is at a disadvantage in their interpersonal communication. A beautiful smile can give a person the kind of self-confidence people recognize immediately. People who were once afraid to smile showing their teeth are now beaming from ear to ear, thanks to the "miracle" of porcelain veneers.

Oral hygiene and gum disease: Of course, there is no substitute for good oral hygiene. By brushing your teeth and flossing daily, you can prevent the onset of adult dental problems. By controlling dental plaque at the gumline and between the teeth, 98 percent of all oral disease can be prevented. Tartar-control toothpaste and anti-plaque mouth rinse do not have the dramatic impact purported in their advertisements.

Most adult tooth loss is the result of periodontal infection, and it is estimated that 75 percent of adults have active periodontal disease. Gingivitis and periodontitis can progress painlessly and rapidly, so it is important to have yourself checked for it. There are many products available to help maintain oral health such as electric toothbrushes, waterjet devices, and even sonic toothbrushes. More important than the tool is the person using it and the diligence with which it is used. The best strategy for fighting the onset of disease is to disrupt the plaque once daily, preferably sometime after dinner and before going to bed. Of course, the best way to ensure yourself a lifetime of healthy and beautiful teeth is to see your dentist regularly and to floss and brush your teeth everyday.

Any time of your life is a prime time for great looks and important challenges. When you look in the mirror at each new phase of your development, you won't see the face of the woman you were in the last transition. But maybe what you see is better, more knowing, more real. And what you see is enhanced if you're eating right and getting good exercise. And your face will be even more beautiful when you own your life experiences with the passing years. Your face can be your billboard to the world. It can show the world you have lived, loved, and laughed. And when you let this kind of energy radiate, it may be a pleasant surprise to find out how much other people will notice. They will be attracted to it. To you. Because you're at peace with who you are. You're not fighting it or hiding it. You're standing tall, as if to say, "I own this ground — I adore who I am."

HEALTHY HABITS

❧

Healthy habits can sound so uninteresting, so boring. Why bother? Isn't life too short? What's the big deal anyway? After all, when will all this drudgery have a payoff? Being stressed-out is just current reality. Live today, diet tomorrow! Exercise next month.

If you have this point of view, it may be hard to convince you otherwise. If you already know the value of a healthy lifestyle, you probably have your eyes on the latest in health news and delight in the rewards of your choice. Could those of you who "just don't feel like trying" to consider thinking about it just for a few minutes? Would it be possible to try just one lifestyle change for three days and be creative enough to make it enjoyable? I like that old quote, "everything in moderation, including moderation," when looking at a new approach to almost anything.

VITAMINS, MINERALS, AND SUPPLEMENTS

Some experts will tell you that healthy eating is the best way to get the vitamins and minerals your body needs. But many women don't have diets that fulfill their nutritional needs. Even a well-designed regimen may not include all the elements you require for optimal health.

For instance, the depletion of estrogen that affects bone strength after menopause makes it difficult for women to get their daily calcium requirements from food and exercise alone. For those who tend to eat few fresh greens, fruits, soy, and grains, and have diets heavy in meat, sauces, pastries, and desserts, supplements will be necessary. However, when you eat well, the advantage of supplements is greatly enhanced.

SOME IMPORTANT VITAMINS AND SUPPLEMENTS TO CONSIDER:

A comprehensive multi-vitamin with trace minerals and antioxidants supports good health and prevents deficiencies. Some reports indicate more people are deficient in minerals than in vitamins. The most familiar antioxidants — vitamins C, E, and betacarotene — are thought to retard the aging process, boost the immune system, and possibly function as anti-cancer agents by protecting against oxidation damage in the DNA. You may need to seek out other nutritional supplements, in addition to your multi-vitamin, to meet your specific requirements.

Vitamin A is essential for normal vision, good cell structure, and healthy skin. It helps to protect the linings of the respiratory, reproductive, digestive, and urinary tracts from infection. Possibly by inhibiting certain chemicals that activate cancer cell growth, it also seems to create barriers to cancer-causing agents.

Vitamin B complex. The full spectrum of B-complex vitamins work together, offering various benefits. They are known for helping with the functioning of the immune system, reducing stress, and balancing moods, as well as metabolizing estrogen. B6, in particular, plays a major role in many of these effects, and B12 is essential for preventing anemia.

Calcium is very important for feeding bones and helping to prevent osteoporosis. Avoid aluminum-based calcium products or those that contain lead. Good sources are chewable antacids tablets with added calcium such as Tums®, Rolaids®, and generic varieties; the highly absorbable calcium citrates for older women; combinations of preferred calcium in the form of capsules; and liquid calcium supplements such as Cal-Mag®. (See the further calcium supplement information in Chapter Five under the discussion about osteoporosis, as well as the Charts in back.)

Vitamin C with bioflavonoids is necessary for many body functions, including building new muscle and bone. Vitamin C is an antioxidant that helps with the immune response to infection, the healing of wounds, and the absorption of iron from the digestive tract. Bioflavonoids are a part of the vitamin C found in natural foods such as citrus pulp and rinds. They help strengthen capillary walls, which may help reduce hot flashes and easy bruising. In some women, they have been known to improve the severity of mood swings.

Vitamin D is needed for healthy bones and teeth. It also aid the absorption of calcium in the intestines and regulation of the body's calcium/phosphate balance.

Vitamin E is useful for healthy, smooth hair and skin and as an antioxidant. A daily dose of 400 to 600 units has been shown to regulate and reduce hot flashes for some women. Vitamin E also can help the heart, although women with high blood pressure, diabetes, and rheumatic heart disease should not take E supplements without consulting their physician.

Flax seed has been recognized as the richest source of valuable omega-3 fatty acids which lower high blood cholesterol and triglyceride levels by as much as 25 percent and 65 percent. The best resource for this is Heintzman Farms, South Dakota, (1-800-333-5813), because their product is impeccably grown.

Iron is a mineral involved in making red blood cells. Supplements may be used for those with iron-deficiency anemia, preoperative patients and those who are pregnant or breast feeding.

Magnesium is indicated for those who have had the

long-term use of diuretics, kidney disorders, or the magnesium deficiency that can come from alcohol abuse. It is also great for calming your mind.

Minerals which contribute to maintaining health are potassium, sodium, calcium, magnesium; and phosphorus. A balanced diet will ordinarily supply the body's mineral needs, but most women need extra calcium to prevent osteoporosis.

Trace elements that are required in small amounts to promote good health are chromium, copper, selenium, sulfur, and zinc.

Which of these, or others, do you need? And how much? Consult with a nutritional specialist, if possible. Linda Prout, M.S., of the Claremont Resort and Spa in Oakland, California, for instance, is one of the most knowledgeable nutritionists you'll find. She publishes an excellent newsletter, *Mind & Energy*. Her philosophy is to "go beyond the nutrition principles you've heard before, to explore leading-edge information." Whatever your resource, try to choose a customized, overall wellness program.

HARMFUL EFFECTS OF STRESS

Stress can be a major contributor to poor health. Stress can adversely affect how you feel, how you look, and how your day goes. It can make you feel nervous, overwhelmed, and irritable. Over time, it can increase the risk of high blood pressure, heart disease, a suppressed immune system, and other major illnesses.

Stress isn't something "out there," it's something in you, inside your body. It's your mind and body's reaction to "something" out there — too much work; not enough time; worry about health, money, children; or even bad traffic.

Our bodies have been equipped with a "fight or flight response," which means the body jumps into action and goes into overdrive unnecessarily, as if it were running away from a flesh-eating monster. This reaction was helpful thousands of years ago when we literally fought off beasts in the woods. But today, those beasts are worry, not enough sleep, unhealthful eating, pressures at work and at home. The list goes on.

Dr. Robert S. Eliot, in his book titled *Is It Worth Dying For?,* has written some of the best advice to date about ways to define and manage the modern-day stress epidemic. Here are some excerpts:

Where stress is concerned, what feels like pressure to one person is stimulation to someone else. Everyone has an individual definition of too much, too little, or just enough stress. That's why there is no objective definition of what a stressful event is or how many events add up to "too much" stress.

Stress is only a burden when you respond to it with the feeling that you have lost control. . . . It is crucial to realize that you can never make everything in the environment go your way. . . . Your own reactions—and over-reactions—are the key. Stress can be the spice of life as well as the kiss of death.

Georgia Witkin, Ph.D., author of *The Female Stress Syndrome,* addresses the unique challenges women face, such as (1) "the stresses of life crises, which fall largely on female shoulders—caring for an ill or dying parent, parenting a child [especially if he or she has major physical and/or emotional difficulties], and making sure that life goes on after divorce in the family;" (2) "the hidden stress of chauvinism, subtle sexism, and infertility;" and (3) "negative attitudes towards a career woman, a mother who works, a mother who doesn't work, an active widow, or an old maid."

Dr. Witkin points out that "whereas men are given serious tests and treatment for their ailments, many physicians still prescribe tranquilizers for women, or tell them, 'Go home and try to relax. Your problem is just stress.'" Meanwhile, special, all-female stresses attack women with "symptoms ranging from loss of menstruation to crippling panic attacks; from transient headaches to life threatening anorexia" or the more familiar "headaches, backaches, erratic menstruation, allergies, colitis, or cardiac arrhythmia."

Most of these symptoms are in response to long-term pressures which are out of your immediate control. Although society's attitudes, family crises, and the pressure of multiple roles are not in your control, how you respond to these stresses is. Remember: take your stresses seriously — the tension you feel today can rob you of your health tomorrow.

Dr. Eliot also offers some poignant remarks about serious stress outcomes:

> *At the lab, I analyzed autopsies of workers who had dropped dead without warning. What I found suggested that adrenaline and other stress chemicals had spewed into their bodies with such strength that they had literally ruptured the muscle fibers of their hearts. It appeared that the brain had the power to trigger heart-stopping emotional reactions to stress. . . .*
>
> *There are many ways you can learn to change your lifestyle and behavior to control the stress in your life so you can be productive without being self-destructive.*

SOME POWERFUL STEPS FOR MANAGING DESTRUCTIVE STRESS:

Avoid harmful triggers. Consuming too much caffeine, chocolate, alcohol, sugar, or tobacco may amplify the "fight or flight" syndrome and add to internal biological stress.

Eat regularly. Stress actually puts a nutritional strain on your body and lowers your immunity, stamina, and estrogen levels. Try smaller, more frequent meals with attention to healthy combinations.

Exercise. Walk around the block. Go out for a brisk morning stroll. Feel your head clear as you put your pressures in perspective.

Learn to breathe. The best remedy for reducing stress at any moment — in your car during a traffic jam, in the dentist's chair, at your desk at work — is to breathe slowly, evenly, deeply for at least a few minutes every hour or so. Good breathing helps your whole body. It relaxes your muscles. It can lower your heart rate. It reduces the stress of the moment. From a health point of view, it is important to learn to breathe with your body, not just your lungs.

BodyBreathing™ is my term for using a breathing movement that involves your lower torso. These are the lowest muscles below your navel that move when you cough or belly laugh. Hold this area with your hands and cough to experience your muscle response. Then to practice BodyBreathing, your lower torso should move out slightly as you breathe in, and inward as you breathe out, the way animals and babies breathe. Repeating this many times throughout the day will help you to become a healthy breather in just a few weeks. You'll find more about relaxation and breathing techniques in my book *Voice Power*, available by calling 1-(800)-820-2010

Take time for yourself. Quiet time. Music. Reading. Listening to stress reduction audio tapes. Whatever turns you on and tunes you in.

Go to seminars. Reputable seminar leaders can teach

you a great deal about how to manage chronic stress patterns.

Seek professional assistance. Various kinds of psychological therapies offered through clinics or practitioners are worth considering. If you find this assis-tance is not easing your symptoms, it may be determined that you need some alternative remedies or medication for your discomfort.

THE OPTIMAL HEALTH ACTION PLAN

Even if you're happy with your current eating and work-out habits, it's great to recognize that there is an "extra mile." Read books, articles, and newsletters about women's health. Buy or rent video and audio tapes. Explore seminars on the subjects that interest you. If time and finances allow, consider these options:

- Speak to an acupuncturist about energy balancing treatments.
- Explore homeopathic remedies for enhancing your immune system and your overall health.
- Ask a nutritionist to customize a vitamin/supplement regimen just for you.
- Choose a chiropractor or osteopath for mobilizing your joints and helping your posture and alignment.
- Try a session with a cranial/sacral professional to balance your overall system. Their work is little known but extremely effective for TMJ problems, headaches, stress, energetic balancing, and general healing.
- Ask a personal trainer to design an exercise program especially for you.
- Consult with a psychologist if you have some unresolved personal agendas.

- Seek out a yoga teacher to learn about relaxation or meditation techniques that will fit into your daily schedule.
- Get a massage specialist whose hands can talk to your muscles, tissues, and ligaments.
- Consider with your health advisor whether you need adrenal supplements to boost your energy.

There's more information than ever before for women. All of us can try to go that extra mile!

WEIGHT ISSUES

WEIGHT LOSS — ESPECIALLY FOR THE FORGOTTEN FEMALE

For health at every age, you hear about the dangers and difficulties associated with weight issues. If you are a thin person, are you automatically a woman with "healthy weight?" Not necessarily. It is just as true that weighing somewhat more than the published "standard" weight is not always unhealthy.

Starting at around age thirty, most females tend to metabolize food at a decrease of about 1 percent each year. The weight gain many experience around menopause is more likely due to the biology of aging rather than hormone replacement therapy, as some have believed.

Women past childbearing who are not on a hormonal regime often find weight gain or weight placement occurring more in the abdominal area than around the hips, buttocks, and thighs. This is normally caused by menopausal hormonal shifts.

For the first time in many years, there is hope for those who have been frustrated or who have given up. Fortunately, some of the stigma of being overweight is shifting, as we realize the extremely difficult barriers to losing weight and maintaining weight loss.

The woman who has always been thin and who gains considerable weight for the first time at menopause deserves the same sensitive, expert attention needed by the woman who has had a lifetime of weight problems.

Sad to say, there are health experts, diet programs, and spas that will tell you that to lose weight all you have to do is eat less and exercise more. Along with that admonition is the almost universal assumption that if you have extra pounds you have unresolved emotional issues or outrageous eating habits. For some this may be true. Yet there are those who eat so little they actually need to eat more calories to activate weight loss.

The important topics of serious eating disorders and food addictions are not covered here. Neither are careless or unconscious eating habits. What I want to share are the highlights of recent discoveries in the study of obesity. Of course, because of the complexity of the subject, there are still many unknowns.

HEALTHY WEIGHT DEFINED

Defining healthy weight is without question the first step needed to approach any other information about weight issues. Deborah Hurlax Durga — an American College of Sports Medicine Certified Health and Fitness Instructor and founder of Designer Fitness in Walnut Creek, California — clarifies what the scale tells us and what it doesn't. She explains body weight versus body composition:

Total body weight or scale weight can be divided into lean and/or fat body mass. "Lean" in this case refers to bone, skin, tissue, muscles, and organs; fat includes fatty tissue.

Body fat ratios to total body weight for women before menopause are considered to be healthy at 18 to 25 percent, and after menopause at 18 to 29 percent. However, the average American woman is in the 35 to 36 percent body fat range, irrespective of total body weight. There are very thin women who have as much as 40 percent or more body fat.

There are various techniques used to determine body composition such as infra-red interactance, dual x-ray absorptionmetry (DEXA), magnetic resonance imaging (MRI), and underwater weighing. Water weighing takes a considerable amount of time and is a bit clumsy. Infra-red interactance is the easiest and least expensive. Since you would most likely get a slightly different reading with each method, it's important to use your choice of measurement consistently over time to determine whether your lean body mass is increasing or decreasing.

New Hope for Losing Pounds

If weight loss programs have not worked for you in the past and you are feeling like giving up, I will have to say that you probably qualify as what I call The Forgotten Female. You could have feelings that you describe as eternally frustrated, always hopeful, self-blaming, ashamed, or guilty. You cannot find the solution for your continually increasing weight gains even after successful losses.

The Forgotten Female may also be someone you know. She is the woman who possibly has an obesity gene, chemical/hormonal imbalances, insulin resistance, seratonin sensitivity, or the inherited tendency to carry more fat pounds than those who have biologically efficient weight regulating capabilities. Or she may have some unbalanced inhibiting factors not yet named.

The Forgotten Female isn't a closet eater, a binger, or a bulimic. She isn't lazy or consuming high-calorie foods morning, noon, and night. Physicians and weight counselors, especially if they're naturally lean, often have little sympathy for her. Empathy or curiosity doesn't come easily for those who haven't been there. The widespread belief is that she could exercise more and eat less. The truth is that she may already be close to clinical exhaustion from over-exercising and malnourished from undereating. It is often assumed she eats more than she says. In fact, her metabolism is just overly efficient in turning food to fat rather than energy.

At menopause our Forgotten Female can become even more frustrated and demoralized. Her changing hormones and changing weight — years of gaining, losing, gaining more — are catching up with her. She can be bloated from medications to curtail menopause symptoms — medications that aren't calibrated for her particular needs. She becomes discouraged. She waits for that surge of extra determination she's always counted on to lose weight one more time. But this time it doesn't surface. She's worn out. The low-fat diet and exercise doesn't work. Not only can't she lose that twenty or thirty or forty pounds that she used to be able to manage, she can't lose anything. Maintaining a weight that is comfortable, age appropriate, and on target, with an 18 to 29 percent body fat in relationship to total body weight should be her goal. Yet other messages abound. Some men, the media, and even best friends frequently want her to attain the "can't be too thin" goal that prevails almost everywhere. Too few clothing designers make wonderful clothes for her.

This woman often has some other traits, as well. She'd rather read a book or see a good film than play tennis, jog, or swim. She feels good before she exercises, but not necessarily any better afterward. She works out because it's healthy for her and possibly will eventually help her lose weight.

Those who get endorphin highs from exercise say she should feel terrific when she gets her heartbeat going and her muscles singing. They assume she's just not adequately willful to keep at it long enough or hard enough. But when she pushes her limit, her energy goes down. She doesn't sweat easily and her blood pressure is on the low side. Humid weather and hot temperatures make her uncomfortable.

When she's working at a good pace physically or mentally, her blood sugar levels drop, and therefore her energy dips down every couple of hours and she needs to eat just to function again. And she's feeling real hunger, not a psychological need. It's better for her to have six small meals a day than three big meals. Unless eaten with a complex carbohydrate or with meals, fruits mess up her energy. The same is true for sugar products.

Phentermine and fenfluramine, also know as the fen/phen, were first used in Europe where they were considered successful, safe, and non-addictive. Michael Weintraub, M.D., was a pioneer in the first major study of these drugs at Rochester Medical Center, and Richard Atkinson, M.D., professor of medicine and nutritional science at the University of Wisconsin, was among the first of those joining in the initial years of clinical testing, prescribing them in combination for safe weight loss. When the drugs were used separately the results were not so encouraging. No adverse side effects were found over an eight-to-ten year period in various practices throughout the country. These medications were released under the names Fastin® or Ionomin® (phentermine) and Pondimin® (fenfluramine).

However, both Pondimin and Redux® — a molecular variant of fenfluramine which was used as a single drug rather than in combination with phentermine — were taken off the market in 1997 because heart valve damage and serious lung conditions were found in a very small but significant group of those using this medication. Studies are underway to find more about why, out of millions of prescriptions, these drugs created serious medical problems for some people.

Sibutramine, brand name Meridia®, gained FDA approval in the fall of 1997 with a release date of March 1998. Tim Seaton, senior medical director at Knoll Pharmaceuticals; says that "unlike the diet drugs taken off the market, sibutramine doesn't boost the release of serotonin, but it increases the amount of time that serotonin and norepinephrine — neurotransmitters involved in controlling appetite — stay between the cells."

Dr. Richard Atkinson asserts that "pharmacology is the future for treating obesity." Yet many doctors aren't aware of the medications currently available and won't consult with the physicians who do, won't consider reviewing the current data, and therefore won't prescribe them. Will power and weight loss programs alone are clearly not the answer for these special cases. On the other hand, medications are not recommended for those individuals who have only five or ten pounds they would like to lose.

The diet drugs that are currently in the FDA approval pipeline include Orlistat, Leptin, OB-Receptor, BTA-243, CCK-Agonist, and NGD-95-1.

Steven Lamm, M.D.—who has a practice in New York City and has just written an excellent book, *Thinner at Last*—advocates not necessarily thin, but healthfully thinner as a goal for his patients. He explains that medications may be the long sought-after solution for certain types of obesity.

Dr. Lamm relays the findings from Jeffrey Friedman, Ph.D., a molecular geneticist who recently discovered a gene related to obesity:

> *The ob gene, which is nearly identical in mouse and human, seems to be switched on in the fat tissue where it generates a hormone-like protein [leptin] that is secreted by the fat cells into the bloodstream. . . . [W]hen the gene is working normally, it helps to regulate weight by sending the brain a hormonal message to stop eating. However, when the gene is mutated or damaged, it either fails to make the proper hormone or it creates an abnormal hormone. As a result, the brain does not receive the message and the individual gains weight. . . . Only time will tell if the key to treating obesity . . . lies in our genes.*

If you are a Forgotten Female, at midlife particularly—but for years before and after as well—you require very special, long-term help. You need a sensitive physician, weight counselor, or nutritional consultant who really understands your inherited biology, as well as your whole behavior/fitness/symptom dynamic. You need someone who has studied this field from the perspective of this story. You may want to contact the American Society of Beriatric Physicians—obesity specialists—in Englewood, Colorado, for names of any clinics, physicians, or specialists in your area.

You will want to consider programs that reflect the very latest research. Read *Mastering the Zone* by Barry Sears,

Ph.D., a pioneer in biotechnology from MIT. He explains certain biochemical tendencies related to weight issues and optimal health that respond well to his customized suggestions about food choices.

Just don't give up. Seek out the answer — whether in the form of medications, supplements, an eating plan, an exercise regimen, or herbal tonics — that's right for you.

Weight problems are a very big business. But it's still a mystery why some people have such trouble holding onto their weight losses when they are exercising, following healthy regimens, and eating for real hunger or needed energy. One theory is the obesity gene behaves in a way to add weight or prevent loss. Pounds are also regained because old eating habits re-emerge and little, if any, exercise is maintained.

To be truly successful, your weight management needs to be individually fine-tuned, just like many other treatments.

We know that the percentage of Americans who are obese has increased by almost 40 percent since the mid-1960s. We know that nine out of ten weight losses do not last. Yet. But it looks like the next decade will offer solutions that in the past were only dreams. Hopefully, if unmanageable weight issues have been your problem, your answer will come soon or be on the near horizon.

SOME CLOSING THOUGHTS

Allow this book to be your guide to optimal wellness. Review the sections that caught your attention. Go through the references and resources that are recommended. And from time to time, be sure to refer to the information, suggestions, and alternatives provided throughout *Whose Body Is It Anyway?*

Take advantage of this book as a resource for a healthier and more informed lifestyle. And as you put on the zesty cloak of an inspired, health-active woman, remember: Know what your options are and be empowered by this knowledge. Choose what is best for you and exult in a new-found confidence. Use the suggestions and choices open to you and take action that will ignite life-affirming results.

The following sections of the book provide essential nutritional information and detail numerous health concerns and treatment options. Fill out a copy of the "Diagnostic Questionnaire" and take it with you to your next physician's appointment. Read through the "Symptoms, Concerns, and Treatment Options" and find answers to questions you may have had for years. Keep track of your medical visits and tests by using the "Check-Up Schedule." Be sure to review the "Food Sources: Vitamin & Mineral Functions" charts for vital information to keep you healthy. And use the references, resources, and other informational pages to remind yourself that the choices are yours, and you are not alone.

PART TWO

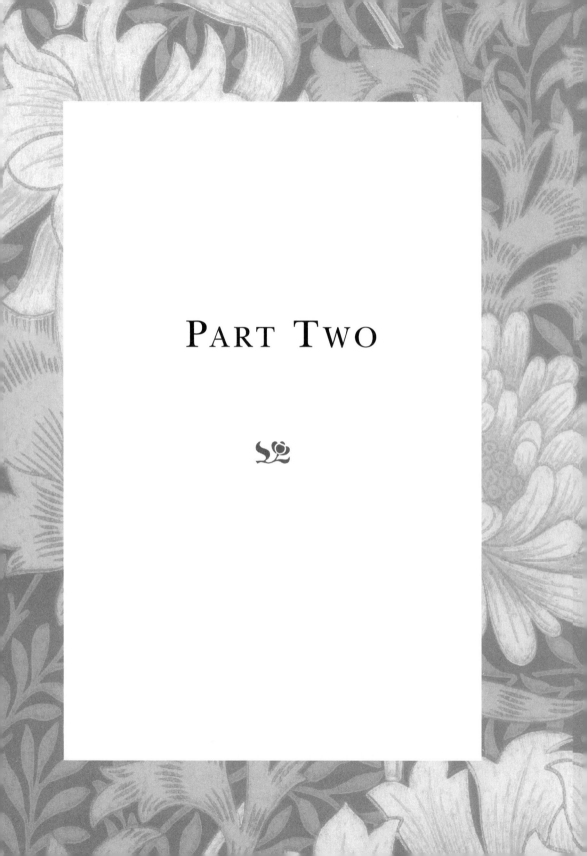

The "Just Do It" Check-Up Schedule

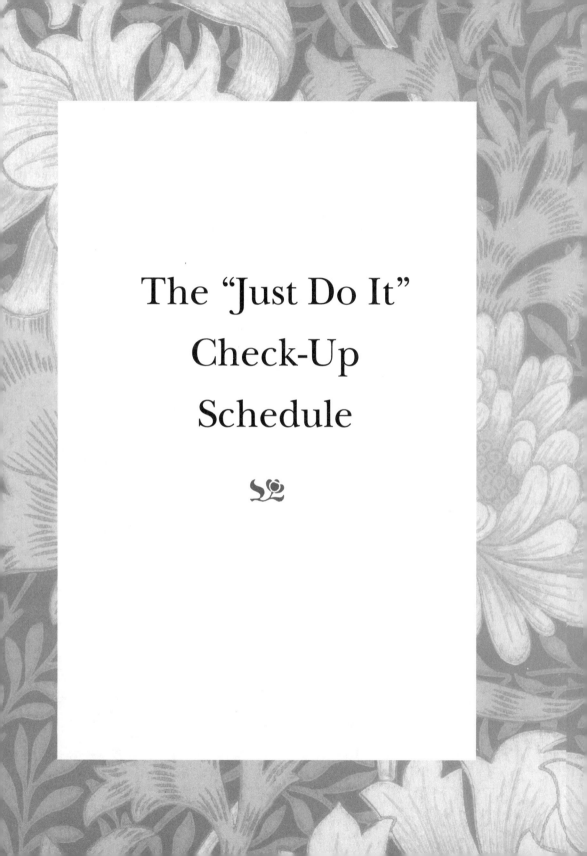

TEST	AGES 35–45	AGES 45–55	AGES 55 & OLDER
Pelvic Exam Physical exam by health advisor to assess for unusual masses and abnormal pain in uterus.	Every year	Every year	Every year
Progesterone Challenge Tests the uterus for excessive buildup of the lining (hyperplasia).	As recommended by health advisor	As recommended by health advisor	As recommended by health advisor
Pelvic-Floor Muscle Evaluates the urine release and/or stop capabilities.	As required for urinary symptoms	As required for urinary symptoms	As required for urinary symptoms

TEST	AGES 35–45	AGES 45–55	AGES 55 & OLDER
Endometrial Tissue Sample Evaluation of the lining of the uterus for cancer or hyperplasia.	6-12 months without a period—with any of the following risk factors: 1. History of infertility 2. Obesity 3. Failure to ovulate 4. Abnormal uterine bleeding 5. On estrogen therapy without progesterone	3-4 months without a period—with any of the following risk factors: 1. History of infertility 2. Obesity 3. Failure to ovulate 4. Abnormal uterine bleeding 5. On estrogen therapy without progesterone	
Pap Smear Detects cancer of the cervix.	Every year	Every year	Every year

TEST	AGES 35–45	AGES 45–55	AGES 55 & OLDER
Complete Blood Chemistry (CBC) Measures hemoglobin concentration and the number of red blood cells, white blood cells and platelets.	As recommended by health advisor	As recommended by health advisor	As recommended by health advisor
Cholesterol (Lipid Profile) Determines blood cholesterol levels for heart disease risk assessment.	Baseline test at age 35, then every 5 years	Every 3 years until menopause, then every other year	Every other year
Diabetes Fasting plasma glucose or urine test of glucose tolerance. Evaluates insulin levels (the hormone responsible for absorption of glucose).	Fasting plasma glucose or dip stick urine test yearly—or as recommended by health advisor	Fasting plasma glucose or dip stick urine test yearly—or as recommended by health advisor	Fasting plasma glucose or dip stick urine test yearly—or as recommended by health advisor

TEST	AGES 35 – 45	AGES 45 – 55	AGES 55 & OLDER
FSH (Follicle Stimulating Hormone) Measures ovary production of estrogen. Can identify women who have reached menopause.	If you have menopausal symptoms **NOTE:** Hormone replacement (HRT) or other remedies may be suggested to women with severe pre-menopausal symptoms even though FSH levels are normal	If you have menopausal symptoms **NOTE:** Hormone replacement (HRT) or other remedies may be suggested to women with severe pre-menopausal symptoms even though FSH levels are normal	
TSH (Thyroid Stimulating Hormone) Regulates metabolism.	As recommended by health advisor	Screen at **45** with TSH assay; annually thereafter	**Until age 60**, with annual physical, **After 60**, every 2 years
Kidney Function Evaluates kidney functioning.	As recommended by health advisor	As recommended by health advisor	As recommended by health advisor

TEST	AGES 35–45	AGES 45–55	AGES 55 & OLDER
Liver Function Evaluates liver functioning.	As recommended by health advisor	As recommended by health advisor	As recommended by health advisor
HIV Detects the human immuno-deficiency virus, which causes AIDS.	Every six months if at high risk or show symptoms of AIDS Annually, if more than one sex partner or as recommended by health advisor	Every six months if at high risk or show symptoms of AIDS Annually, if more than one sex partner or as recommended by health advisor	Every six months if at high risk or show symptoms of AIDS Annually, if more than one sex partner or as recommended by health advisor
Sex Hormones Evaluates male (andro-gen) and female (estro-gen and progesterone) sex hormone levels.	As recommended by health advisor	As recommended by health advisor	As recommended by health advisor

TEST	AGES 35–45	AGES 45–55	AGES 55 & OLDER
Blood Pressure Evaluates the "pressure" in the vascular tube.	With every exam (or once a year) or as recommended by health advisor	With every exam (or once a year) or as recommended by health advisor	With every exam (or once a year) or as recommended by health advisor
Exercise Stress Test Measures oxygen consumption.	As indicated by symptoms or medical history	As indicated by symptoms or medical history	As indicated by symptoms or medical history

TEST	AGES 35–45	AGES 45–55	AGES 55 & OLDER
Echo-cardiogram (Sonogram of the Heart) Ultrasound used to obtain an image of the heart for detection of structural, and some functional abnormalities of the heart wall, valves and the blood vessels.	As indicated by symptoms or medical history	As recommended by health advisor	As recommended by health advisor
Electro-cardiogram (EKG or ECG) Measures the electrical activity in the heart.	As indicated by symptoms or medical history	As indicated by symptoms or medical history	As indicated by symptoms or medical history

244

TEST	AGES 35 – 45	AGES 45 – 55	AGES 55 & OLDER
Weight and Body Composition Skin Fold Girth measurements DEXA (Dual Energy X-Ray Absorptionometry) Used to identify women who are at risk due to body weight/body composition problems.	For all women — if there's any question about body weight composition	For all women — if there's any question about body weight composition	For all women — if there's any question about body weight composition
DEXA (Dual Energy X-Ray Absorptionometry) Measures bone width and the condition of the bones.	DEXA tests at age **35**, then every 3-5 years or as recommended by health advisor	If indicated by urine test, every 3 years until menopause, then every year or as recommended by health advisor; otherwise a baseline DEXA at age **50** if NOT on HRT	Every year or as recommended by health advisor

TEST	AGES 35–45	AGES 45–55	AGES 55 & OLDER
Crown-to-Rump Height Used to measure a loss of stature, fractures of the vertebrae and osteoporosis.	Every 5 years	Every 5 years	Every year
Vaginal and Uterine Ultrasound For vaginal or abdominal cancer detection or to check the endometrial lining in the uterus (as recommended by health advisor after a physical exam).	As recommended by health advisor or if any of the following exist: 1. Two or more first-order relatives who have had ovarian cancer 2. Presence of a palpable pelvic mass 3. Abnormal uterine bleeding 4. Pelvic discomfort and abdominal distention if related to suspicion of cancer	As recommended by health advisor or if any of the following exist: 1. Two or more first-order relatives who have had ovarian cancer 2. Pelvic discomfort 3. Abdominal distention 4. Presence of a palpable pelvic mass 5. Abnormal uterine bleeding	As recommended by health advisor or if any of the following exist: 1. Two or more first-order relatives who have had ovarian cancer 2. Pelvic discomfort 3. Abdominal distention 4. Presence of a palpable pelvic mass 5. Abnormal uterine bleeding

TEST	AGES 35–45	AGES 45–55	AGES 55 & OLDER
Serum CA 125 levels For ovarian cancer detection. As of this writing, the helpfulness of this test is unknown. **NOTE:** To date, these tests have not decreased mortality rates.			
Breast Self-Exam For identification of unusual lumps or masses that should be brought to the attention of a health advisor. Eighty-five percent of all lump detections are found by women who self-exam.	Check monthly or more frequently if recommended by health advisor	Check monthly or more frequently if recommended by health advisor	Check monthly or more frequently if recommended by health advisor

TEST	AGES 35–45	AGES 45–55	AGES 55 & OLDER
Breast Exam by Health Advisor For detection of cancerous changes in breast tissue.	Every year	Every year	Every year
Mammogram For early detection of breast lumps that are too small to be discovered by self-exam or health advisor exam.	Baseline test at **35 or 40** based on health advisor's recommendation	**40-50 years** With risk factors, every 1 to 2 years or as recommended by health advisor **50-60 years** Every year	Every year
Skin Exam For detection of skin abnormalities or cancer.	Self-exam: monthly Health advisor exams: 1. **Before age 40,** every 3 years 2. **After age 40,** every year	Self-exam: monthly Health advisor exams: every year	Self-exam: monthly Health advisor exams: every year

TEST	AGES 35 – 45	AGES 45 – 55	AGES 55 & OLDER
Digital Rectal Exam Used to check for prolapsed rectum, hemorrhoids or abnormalities that signal early signs of colon cancer.	Every year	Every year	Every year
Stool Test (Occult or Hidden Blood) Used for evaluation and early detection of colon cancer.	Every year	Every year	Every year
Flexible Sigmoidoscopy Examination of lower part of colon for abnormalities that signal early signs of colon cancer.	As recommended by health provider if you have symptoms or high risk profile	**Over 50** every 3-5 years	Every 3-5 years

TEST	AGES 35–45	AGES 45–55	AGES 55 & OLDER
Colonoscopy Checks upper part of colon not seen by sigmoidoscopy.	With significant risk factors for colon cancer	With significant risk factors for colon cancer	With significant risk factors for colon cancer
Chest X-RAY (Lung) Used to detect advanced stage lung cancer.	As recommended by health advisor if any of the following risk factors exist: 1. Persistent cough 2. Bloody sputum 3. Chest pain 4. Recurring pneumonia or bronchitis	As recommended by health advisor if any of the following risk factors exist: 1. Persistent cough 2. Bloody sputum 3. Chest pain 4. Recurring pneumonia or bronchitis	As recommended by health advisor if any of the following risk factors exist: 1. Persistent cough 2. Bloody sputum 3. Chest pain 4. Recurring pneumonia or bronchitis

TEST	AGES 35 – 45	AGES 45 – 55	AGES 55 & OLDER
General Health Appraisal and Risk Assessment Personal and family medical history, lifestyle inventory, pre-existing conditions; to assess risk for:	1. Breast disease 2. Cancer 3. Osteoporosis 4. Vascular disease 5. Heart disease risk 6. Risk of stroke	1. Breast disease 2. Cancer 3. Osteoporosis 4. Vascular disease 5. Heart disease risk 6. Risk of stroke	1. Breast disease 2. Cancer 3. Osteoporosis 4. Vascular disease 5. Heart disease risk 6. Risk of stroke
Health Counseling To provide information about: 1. Smoking 2. Sun exposure 3. Diet and nutrition 4. Sexuality issues 5. Environmental and other occupational exposures	As needed	As needed	As needed

Test	Ages 35–45	Ages 45–55	Ages 55 & Older
Dental Checkup Regular dental check-ups; after menopause, possible bone loss in jaws and loss of teeth without ERT.	Every 6 months or as recommended by dentist or other health advisor	Every 6 months or as recommended by dentist or other health advisor	Every 6 months or as recommended by dentist or other health advisor
Eye Exam To detect glaucoma, cataracts or declining vision.	Every 1-2 years or as recommended by health advisor	Every 1-2 years or as recommended by health advisor	Every 1-2 years or as recommended by health advisor
Hearing Exam For hearing loss detection.	As recommended by health advisor	As recommended by health advisor	As recommended by health advisor

Know Your Alternative
Treatment Options

❧

*A*lternative/complementary and standard therapies are mentioned throughout this book as treatment choices. Inasmuch as standard Western medicine is familiar to almost everyone, you'll find some definitions of the alternative/complementary healing practices below. In general, a majority of these methods are about keeping you well, balancing your mind/body system, easing or curing chronic conditions, reducing pain, and enhancing structural problems. The guiding purpose is to treat causes, not just symptoms. One-third of all patients in this country report seeking nontraditional treatments; on an unreported basis, there are many more.

Alternative options are often incorporated into the standard Western medical practices that commonly treat countless conditions and acute diseases through medication and surgeries. Sometimes non-Western therapies act as the primary treatment source for major illnesses. When dealing with serious health concerns, you have to choose for yourself — using reliable information — which discipline will serve your healing as well as inspire your faith and confidence. When appropriate, you might consider a combination of traditions rather than an "either/or" approach.

The following list may stimulate your thinking about exploring non-traditional therapies. (It is not intended to imply any exclusion of standard medical procedures or practitioners.)

Acupuncture. Fine, sterilized needles are inserted into the body at points along the meridians through which the qi (chi) or vital energy flows. The needles help to create a balanced energy in the system by using the specific acupoints on the body that stimulate the release of healing vital energy. Acupuncture also uses other methods besides the insertion of needles: electronic devices that beam energy to the site; small pellets that can be taped on like a small bandage; tiny, short needles that can be inserted into your ear to wear for a designated period of time; and moxibustion — burning, healing herbs held near the acupoint.

Alpha-Stim 100. This device delivers a different type and a more effective low-grade electrical stimulus compared to the traditional TENS, and is producing impressive results in pain control. In addition to relieving chronic and short term pain, physicians report that some patients experience a decrease in anxiety and depression.

Aromatherapy. Essential herbs and fragrances are used in oils and creams to soothe, relieve, or heal allergies, emotional states, and physical discomfort.

Alexander Technique. Reeducating the body, through various exercises, deep breathing, and realignment, to correct unhealthy posture as well as improve function and coordination of the body, mind, and voice.

Ayurveda. Five thousand years old, this methodology focuses on the prevention of disease. Ayurveda functions on the dosha principles of vata, pitta, and kapha that identify a person's physical, emotional, mental, and spiritual qualities. Each individual has a particular combination of doshas, and this indicates the flow of that individual's "life force" throughout the body. The techniques involved address physical fitness, eating habits, and choices related to the seasons, home/work/social environments, and any other lifestyle behavior that affects your overall health.

Biofeedback. Small electronic equipment is used to observe subtle changes in body heat, muscle reactions, heart rhythms, and other physical reactions. When a person's awareness is heightened, techniques are taught to create positive responses without the equipment so that clients can eventually self-manage the problem.

Bodywork. Various hands-on healing and pain-relieving therapies fall into this category. They are known for improving the circulation, enhancing the nerve and lymphatic systems, stretching and soothing muscles, and promoting body/mind relaxation. Some of these body therapies include:

Craniosacral Therapy. The gentle adjustment of the sutures of the skull bones helps to balance the alignment of the skull as well as enhance the flow of spinal fluid. This work has positive effects on the autonomic nervous system, TMJ problems, chronic pain, ear pain, and headaches.

Chinese Medicine. Chinese doctors use what they see, hear, smell, and touch when observing a patient from both a physical and an emotional perspective. Most importantly, they are skilled in diagnostic observation of the tongue and sensitive evaluation of the wrist pulse. There are twelve positions to check on the wrist with twenty-eight types of pulses at each site. Through this methodology, a practitioner can diagnose what illnesses may be developing up to five years before the disease is apparent. Therefore, much of this work is very beneficial for prevention, though it is used for treatment as well.

This technique of promoting wellness is based on the quality of the qi and how it affects each organ in the body. The philosophy contends that the passive yin and active yang forces must be balanced or an individual will be susceptible to various diseases. The six external causative factors for Chinese medicine are cold, dryness, dampness, heat, summer heat, and wind. The theory is that infection, bad nutrition, and too much stress interact with the six external factors to create illness. However, it has been said that once a disease has developed, Western medicine may be the better choice for diagnosing the ailment.

Acupuncture, moxibustion, herbal remedies, and other procedures are used along with a variety of suggestions about behavior and diet.

Chiropractic. The muscular and skeletal structures of the body are manipulated to re-align and release areas that are causing difficulty. Some disciplines adjust the neck or the complete spine only, while others adjust any joint and structural dysfunction in the body. Sometimes soft and deep tissue and muscle massage are included in the treatment. Ice packs, heat packs, ultrasound treatments, and electronic muscle stimulation are not uncommon during the sessions. The goal is to improve and heal structural problems, chronic pain, muscle spasms, and other complaints by viewing the body as a total health system. Paralleling internal hormonal change, women tend to have an increase in aching muscles and joint stiffness. After thirty-five — and more specifically after menopause — muscle and skeletal stress from previous injuries, surgeries, emotional holding patterns, etc., can have a compounding effect.

There can be difficulty maintaining an exercise program due to structural, biochemical, and/or functional instability. Chiropractic and osteopathic manual manipulative techniques, along with personalized strengthening and flexibility exercises, can often solve these problems.

Feldenkrais Method. A system of specifically designed exercises and breathing techniques meant to improve an individual's tension and movement patterns that have become unconscious negative habits in daily life.

Guided Imagery. A trainer teaches the client to visualize specific images in the mind that will aid in fighting disease, strengthening the immune system, and managing pain and relaxation. Dr. Carl Simonton pioneered many of these techniques in cancer treatment while continuing the use of standard medical practices.

Herbal Remedies. Please note: when personally considering over-the-counter herbal supplements that are not specifically recommended by a reputable health advisor, be aware that the products may not provide what is claimed on the labels and the active ingredients from one brand to another may vary considerably. For instance, Consumer Reports tested ten brands of ginseng, and the active ingredient was twenty times greater in the most potent brand than in the brand with the least potency. The November 1995 issue stated: "These products don't have to be tested for safety or effectiveness as conventional drugs are. So it's hard to know just what's in the supplements take, and whether they might help you or harm you . . . . [Some] may be downright dangerous."

However, properly prescribed, herbal remedies can be extremely helpful and healing.

Homeopathy. Samuel Christian Hahnemann, M.D., founded this practice in the early eighteenth century. Homeopathy asserts that symptoms are the body's natural defense mechanism. The theory is that if a healthy person is given a certain substance that causes specific reactions, then that very substance — in tiny doses — will be curative for a patient who has an illness presenting those same symptoms. Homeopathic remedies are diluted in alcohol or distilled water. They are also available in very small pellets that are dissolved under the tongue. Books can be found detailing many remedies that are available at health food stores. However, a homeopathic physician can prescribe stronger substances that usually don't require lengthy therapy. There are certain foods and medications that are not compatible when taking homeopathic treatments. When prescribed by a professional, each remedy is personalized according to the practitioner's trained observation of the patient's mind, body, and emotional traits, as well as a detailed personal history.

Massage. There are more varieties of massage now than ever before. They can relax, rejuvenate, release, and refresh. Some types are Swedish, Esalen, California, sports, deep tissue, shiatsu, acupressure, lymphatic drainage, and body strengthening through resistance techniques.

Music Therapy. French physician Alfred Tomatis's research inspired author Don Campbell to write about music's direct impact on health, creativity, and mental strength in *The Mozart Effect.* For example, music is being used at The Listening and Learning Center in Phoenix, Arizona, to treat people with adult attention deficit disorder, speech problems, autism, symptoms of a stroke, and fatigue. Although Campbell hails Mozart's music as the best all around assistant, he suggests the following: Gregorian chants to create a sense of spaciousness for meditation and relaxation; baroque music (Bach, Handel, Vivaldi) to create a mental environment good for study or work; impressionist music (Debussy, Ravel, Faure) to unlock your creative impulses and tap into your unconscious; and sacred music (shamanic drumming, gospel music, church hymns) to help you transcend and release pain.

Naturopathy. Referred to as "alternative medicine's general practitioners," naturopaths use any field of alternative medicine that will accommodate the diagnosis. Their intention is to choose treatments that do not cause negative reactions or risks to the body; they address the energy of healing that is innate in everyone from the broad consideration of mental, emotional, physical, and spiritual perspectives.

Nikken Magnetic Therapy. Relatively new in the United States, this is an internationally patented magnetic healing system, using products with concentric circles of North and South polarity. Use of these polarized magnets in the form of mattresses, wrist bands, chair/car seats, pads, etc. re-creates the body's natural magnetic field. They have been known to improve circulation and lymphatic drainage, relieve muscle tightness/spasms, joint and arthritis pain, and headaches, as well as enhance sleep and improve other conditions.

Prayer. Dr. Larry Dossey's book, *Healing Words: The Power of Prayer & The Practice of Medicine,* offers an in-depth and impressive account of prayer and its role in recovery from illness — a truly significant consideration that science and medicine do not always choose to recognize. There is increasing awareness among many, however, that the healing potential of the spiritual can be a compelling force in both curing disease and maintaining wellness.

Reiki. Developed two centuries ago by a Buddhist monk, this method involves healing a person's subtle energies and, in some circumstances, leading one to transcend ego contractions. Practitioners, who have been trained in specific techniques, work with their hands on or just above the body. Treatment is non-invasive.

Relationships in Healing. There are countless healing possibilities found in the loving care and interaction of friends, partners, relatives, family, and support groups. Many studies reveal the positive dynamic of "someone or something to live for" in the accounts of recovery. This theory extends to beloved hobbies, plants, and animals.

Rolfing. Uses deep massage to release pent-up emotions stored in the body as muscular tension. The intention is to bring balanced alignment to the body and stimulate wellness.

The Rosen Method. By following subtle changes in muscle tension and shifts in breath, practitioners guide people with words and touch to recognize what has been stored in their unconscious muscle tension. This information can encourage people to make choices based on authentic internal experiences.

Shiatsu. This is a Japanese healing method reflecting the philosophy of Traditional Chinese Medicine. It encompasses various aspects: the therapeutic massage of Japan, using finger pressure on the acupuncture points that occur along the body's twelve meridians or energy lines; meditation; self-healing consciousness; and an energetic interaction between the practitioner and client. The intention is to free any blocked vital energy (*qi, chi, ki*) so that it can circulate naturally.

Therapeutic Touch. Begun by ancient Greek physicians, trained individuals use a laying-on of hands technique to exchange life force energies. Energy is directed for the express purpose of healing. It helps people who may feel out of balance, vaguely ill, or continually fatigued, as well as helping to heal the remnants of old injuries or past disease. Used frequently as a complementary option to medical treatment, during operations for enhanced recovery, or when traditional medical intervention has not provided satisfactory results.

259

Vegetarian diets, nutritional programs, juice regimes, meditation, Qigong, Tai Chi, yoga, iridology, healing circles, and mind/body emotional therapies (e.g., Reichian and Bioenergetic work) are other valuable disciplines and therapies to consider, among others not listed here.

❧

Miracles of healing happen every day, often in ways that are inexplicable and mysterious. The open attitude that is necessary for exploring alternatives in health care can lead to amazing and powerful discoveries.

In exploring alternatives, we must not leave Western medicine aside. There must be balance. The mind does give the body messages. Yet we must not blame every illness and physical lapse on our thoughts, behavior, feelings, and perceptions. That attitude would only lay the groundwork for unhealthy personal guilt and unnecessary emotional suffering.

The Heart of
Nourishment

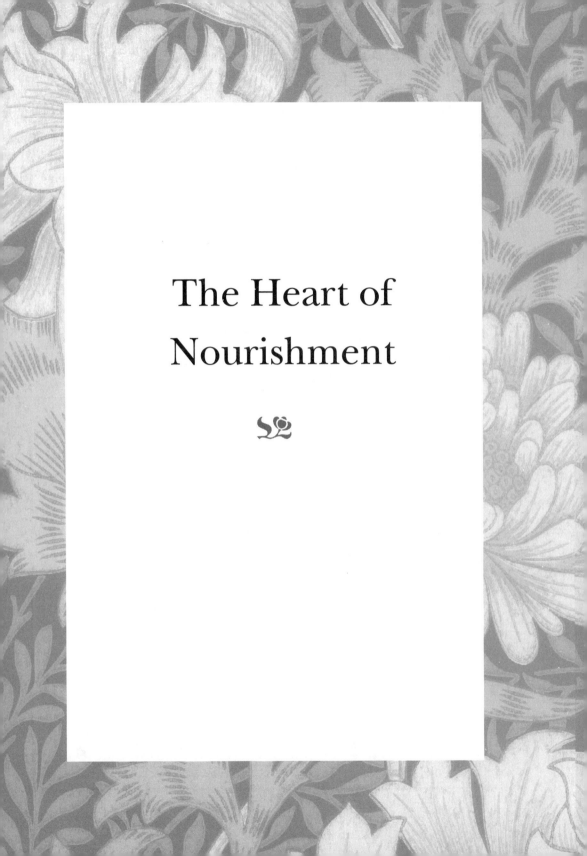

PRODUCE NUTRITION CHART

VEGETABLES, RAW	Total calories	Protein	Carbohydrates	Total fat	Fiber	Sodium	% U.S. RDA			
	cal	g	g	g	g	mg	Vitamin A	Vitamin C	Calcium	Iron
ASPARAGUS, 5 spears (3.5oz/93g)	18	2	2	0	2	0	10	10	*	*
BELL PEPPER, 1 medium (5.5oz/148g)	25	1	5	1	2	0	2	130	*	*
BROCCOLI, 1 medium stalk (5.5oz/148g)	40	5	4	1	5	75	10	240	*	4
CABBAGE, GREEN, 1/2 medium head (3oz/85g)	18	1	3	0	2	30	*	70	6	*
CARROT, 1 medium (7" long, 1 1/2" diameter) (3oz/78g)	40	1	8	1	1	40	330	8	4	*
CAULIFLOWER, 1/8 medium head (5.5oz/148g)	18	2	3	0	2	45	*	110	2	2
CELERY, 2 medium stalks (4oz/110g)	20	1	4	0	2	140	*	15	2	*
CORN, SWEET, kernels from 1 medium ear (3oz/85g)	75	3	17	1	1	15	5	10	4	3
CUCUMBER, 1/3 medium (3.5oz/99g)	18	1	3	0	0	0	4	6	*	2
GREEN BEAN, SNAP, 3/4 C cut (3oz/85g)	14	1	2	0	3	0	3	8	2	*
GREEN ONION, 1/4 chopped (1oz/25g)	7	0	1	0	0	0	2	20	4	5
LETTUCE, ICEBERG, 1/6 medium head (3oz/85g)	20	1	4	0	1	10	20	4	*	*
LETTUCE, LEAF, 1 1/2 cups shredded (3oz/85g)	12	1	1	0	1	40	*	4	*	*
MUSHROOM, 5 medium (3oz/85g)	25	3	3	0	0	0	*	2	4	*
ONION, 1 medium (5.5oz/148g)	60	1	14	0	3	10	*	20	*	*
POTATO, 1 medium (5.5oz/148g)	110	3	23	0	3	10	*	50	4	8
RADISH, 7 radishes (3oz/85g)	20	0	3	0	0	35	*	30	*	*
SQUASH, SUMMER, 1/2 medium (3.5oz/99g)	20	1	3	0	1	0	4	25	2	2
SWEET POTATO, 1 medium 5" long, 2" diameter (4.5oz/130g)	140	2	32	0	3	15	520	50	3	4
TOMATO, 1 medium (5.5oz/148g)	35	1	6	1	1	10	20	40	*	2

Data Source: Nutrition Labeling Data Provided by Food and Drug Administration.
* Contains less than 2% of U.S. RDA

VITAMIN A	BETA CAROTENE (Converts to Vitamin A)	BIOTIN	B1 (THIAMIN)
Dairy milk eggs cheese butter **Fruits** apricot avocado mango cantaloupe papaya peach persimmon **Meat, Poultry, Seafood** crab halibut liver - all types mackerel salmon swordfish **Oils** fish oil **Vegetables** broccoli carrot carrot juice collard greens dandelion greens green onions kale mustard greens parsley spinach sweet potatoes turnip greens winter squash yellow and dark green vegetables	**Fruits** apricots avocado cantaloupe mangos peaches pink grapefruits **Vegetables** broccoli carrots chard collard greens kale leafy greens mustard greens red bell peppers spinach sweet potatoes yams tomatoes winter squash	**Dairy** eggs milk **Fruits** bananas **Grains** brewer's yeast whole grains **Meat, Poultry, Seafood** liver **Vegetables** mushrooms tomatoes	**Fruit** citrus fruit **Vegetables** asparagus cauliflower cabbage kale **Seaweed** assorted **Grains** bran brewer's yeast enriched grain products pasta wheat germ whole grains

B1
(cont.)

Meat, Poultry, Seafood
fish
liver
pork
red meat

Herbal Sources
peppermint
burdock
sage
yellow dock
alfalfa
red clover
fenugreek
raspberry leaves
nettles
catnip
watercress
yarrow
rosehips

B2
(RIBOFLAVIN)

Dairy
dairy products
eggs
milk

Grains
brewer's yeast
enriched grain
  products
cereals
pasta

Legumes
dried beans

Meat, Poultry, Seafood
chicken
fish
liver
organ meat
poultry
red meat

Nuts & Seeds
almonds

Seaweeds
assorted

Vegetables
dried peas
dark, leafy
  greens
onions
mushrooms

Herbal Sources
alfalfa
dandelion
dulse
echinacea
ginseng
hops
kelp
nettles
parsley
peppermint
rosehips
yellow dock

B3
(NIACIN)

Dairy
dairy products

Grains
whole grains
enriched grain
  products

Meat, Poultry, Seafood
chicken
fish
lean meat
liver
poultry
red meat
tuna

Nuts & Seeds
nuts
peanut butter

B3 (Cont.)	B5 (Pantothenic Acid)	B6 (Pyroxidine)	B12
Vegetables asparagus cabbage **Herbal Sources** alfalfa echinacea hops licorice nettles parsley raspberry leaf red clover rosehips slippery elm	**Dairy** egg yolks milk **Grains** whole grains **Legumes** beans **Meat, Poultry, Seafood** liver organ meats poultry **Nuts & Seeds** nuts **Vegetables** dark leafy greens	**Fruits** avocados bananas cantaloupe prunes **Grains** brewer's yeast whole grains wheat germ **Legumes** dried beans lentils **Nuts & Seeds** nuts	**Meat, Poultry, Seafood** beef chicken fish liver poultry red meat **Vegetables** broccoli dark green, leafy vegetables potatoes	**Dairy** cheese eggs milk yogurt **Grains** fortified cereals legumes soy products **Meat, Poultry, Seafood** beef liver pork poultry shellfish

VITAMIN C

Fruits
blackberries
blackcurrants
cantaloupe
citrus fruits
elderberries
grapefruits
grapefruit juice
guava
kiwi fruit
mango
melons
oranges
orange juice
pineapples
raspberries
strawberries
tangerines

Vegetables
asparagus
broccoli
Brussel sprouts
cabbage
cauliflower
collard greens
green onions
green peas
kale
kohlrabi
leafy greens
parsley
potatoes
rutabaga
sweet peppers
sweet potatoes
tomatoes
turnips

Legumes
black-eyed peas

**Meat, Poultry,
Seafood**
liver - all types
pheasant
quail
salmon

Herbal Sources
alfalfa
dandelion greens
echinacea
hops
nettles
raspberry leaf
red clover
rosehips
skullcap
yellow dock root

CALCIUM

Dairy
buttermilk
cheddar cheese
cottage cheese
eggs
nonfat milk
nonfat yogurt

Fruits
blackberries
blackcurrants
blueberries
boysenberries
dates
oranges
papayas
pineapple juice
prunes
raisins
rhubarb
tangerines

Grains
bran
brown rice
bulgar
millet
whole wheat
bread

Seaweeds
agar
hiziki
kelp
kombu
wakame

VITAMIN D
(CHOLECALCIFEROL)

Dairy
butter
eggs
milk

Oils
cod liver oil
fish oil

Meat, Poultry, Seafood
herring
liver
mackerel
salmon
sardines
shrimp
tuna

CALCIUM
(cont.)

Legumes
black beans
black-eyed peas
garbanzo beans
kidney beans
lentils
pinto beans
soybeans
soy milk
tofu

Nuts & Seeds
almonds
sesame seeds
sesame seed
  products

Other
molasses

Vegetables
artichokes
beet greens
broccoli
brussel sprouts
cabbage
chard
collards
eggplant
green beans
green onions
kale
leeks
mustard greens
parsley
parsnips
rutabaga
spinach
turnip greens
watercress

Meat, Poultry, Seafood
abalone
beef
bluefish
carp
cod
crab
haddock
herring
lamb
lobster
oysters
sardines
perch
salmon
shrimp
venison

Herbal Sources
amaranth leaf
borage
chickweed
comfrey
dandelion greens
horsetail
lamb's quarter
mustard greens
nettles
oat straw
peppermint
red clover
sage
uva ursi
valerian
yellow dock

267

FOLIC ACID

Vegetables
asparagus
beets
broccoli
carrots
dark, leafy
  greens
romaine lettuce
spinach
Swiss chard

Fruits
citrus fruits &
  juices

Grains
brewer's yeast
wheat germ
whole grains

Legumes
dried beans & peas
soybeans

**Meat, Poultry,
Seafood**
liver
kidneys

Herbal Sources
alfalfa
chickweed
comfrey leaves
nettles
parsley
peppermint
sage

VITAMIN E (TOCOPHEROL)

Fruits
mangos

Grains
brown rice
millet
wheat germ
whole grains

**Meat, Poultry,
Seafood**
haddock
herring
mackerel
lamb
liver - all types

Nuts & Seeds
almonds
brazil nuts
hazelnuts
peanuts
raw seeds

Oils
cold-pressed oils
corn oil
peanut oil
safflower oil
sesame oil
soybean oil
wheat germ oil

Vegetables
asparagus
cabbage
cucumber
dark, leafy greens
green peas
kale
olives

Herbal Sources
alfalfa
dandelion
don quai
nettles
rosehips
watercress

Iron

Dairy
eggs

Fruits
apricots
dates
prune juice
raisins
strawberries

Grains
bran
brown rice
cornmeal
oats
wheat germ
whole grains

Legumes
kidney beans
lentils
lima beans
peas
soybeans

Nuts & Seeds
sunflower seeds

Seaweed
assorted

Vegetables
asparagus
beets
beet greens
broccoli
potato
spinach
turnip greens
winter squash

Other
molasses

Meat, Poultry, Seafood
beef
chicken
clams
lamb
liver
hamburgers
oysters
pork
sardines
shrimp
turkey

Herbs
black cohosh
burdock
chickweed
dandelion
 root/leaf
don quai
echinacea
horsetail
licorice
milk thistle seed
nettles
peppermint
uva ursi
valerian
yellow dock
Floradex Iron
 w/herbs

Vitamin K

Dairy
eggs
milk
yogurt
legumes
soybeans
soy products

Meat, Poultry, Seafood
liver

Seaweed
kelp

Vegetables
broccoli
brussel sprouts
cabbage
cauliflower
leafy greens
peas

Other
blackstrap
molasses

Herbal Sources
alfalfa
green tea
kelp
nettles

MAGNESIUM

Dairy
cheese
yogurt

Fruits
bananas
grapefruit juice
papaya
pineapple juice
prunes
raisins

Grains
millet
rice, brown and
wild

Legumes
black-eyed peas
green peas
lima beans
soybean sprouts

Nuts & Seeds
almonds
brazil nuts
hazelnuts
peanuts
pistachios

Vegetables
artichokes
avocados
carrot juice
corn
leafy greens
leeks
okra
parsnips
peas
potatoes
spinach
squash
yams

Herbal Sources
burdock
chickweed
dandelion greens
evening primrose
horsetail
licorice
nettles
oat straw
raspberry leaf
red clover
sage
valerian
yellow dock

Meat, Poultry, Seafood
beef
carp
clams
cod
chicken
crab
duck
haddock
herring
lamb
lobster
mackerel
oysters
salmon
shrimp
snapper
turkey

MAGNESIUM
(Cont.)

Grains
wheat germ
bran
whole grains

Nuts & Seeds
sesame seeds

SELENIUM

Seafood
herring
tuna

Herbal Sources
black cohosh
echinacea
ginseng
hawthorn berries
hops
milk thistle
raspberry leaf
rosehips
uva versi
valerian
yellow dock

Fruits
apricots
blackberries
blueberries
cantaloupe
cranberries
dates
figs
grapefruits
grapes
honeydew
lemons
nectarines
oranges
peaches
pears
pineapple
prunes
raspberries
strawberries
tangerines
watermelon

Grains
buckwheat
cornstarch
millet
tapioca
unenriched white
flour products
white rice,
unenriched

Legumes
peas
beans (must be
immature)

Nuts & Seeds
flaxseed
spices
celery powder
onion powder
sweet basil
sweet dill
thyme
vanilla

Vegetables
asparagus
beets
broccoli
Brussels sprouts
cabbage
cauliflower
celery
cucumbers
greens (all)
lettuce
okra
onions
parsnips
pumpkin
radishes
rhubarb
rutabagas
squash
turnips

Animal Products
all meats
cheese
cottage cheese
eggs
milk
yogurt

Fruits
apples
cherries
coconut
olives
plums

Grains
all cereals (except
rye, buckwheat
and white rice)
wheat germ

Legumes
calabar beans
peanuts
soy products

Vegetables
carrots
eggplant
peppers
potatoes
tomatoes
yams

CALCIUM RICH FOODS

FOOD	AMOUNT	MGS CALCIUM	CALORIES
DAIRY			
Yogurt, lowfat plain	1 Cup	415	145
Yogurt, nonfat	1 Cup	271	110
Lowfat milk (2%)	1 Cup	297	120
Nonfat milk (1%)	1 Cup	300	100
Skim milk	1 Cup	302	85
Whole milk	1 Cup	291	150
Buttermilk	1 Cup	300	100
Nonfat instant milk	1 Cup	836	244
Lowfat soy milk	1 Cup	80	72
Mozzarella (skim milk)	1 Ounce	207	80
Lowfat cottage cheese	1 Cup	150	180
Skim ricotta cheese	1 Cup	670	340
DESSERTS			
Nonfat frozen yogurt	1 Cup	272	200
Nonfat ice cream	1 Cup	194	180

NOTE: Cheese is a calcium-rich food which is often too high in fat to recommend to women 50 years and older (because of the increased risk of heart disease associated with high-saturated fat diets).

Calcium Rich Foods

Food	Amount	Mgs Calcium	Calories
Fruits			
Orange	1 Medium	55	70
Apple	1 Medium	10	85
Grains			
Whole wheat bread	1 Slice	20	70
Cooked spaghetti	1 Cup	15	215
Cooked rice	1 Cup	20	160
Meat, Poultry, Seafood			
Sardines with bones	4 Ounces	490	225
Salmon with bones, canned	4 Ounces	220	140
Chum salmon	4 Ounces	365	135
Coho salmon (canned)	4 Ounces	365	185
Pink humpback salmon	4 Ounces	290	132
Chicken	4 Ounces	13	187
Tuna	4 Ounces	7	147
Hamburger patty	4 Ounces	13	300
Egg	1 Large	30	90
Oysters	1 Cup	160	226
Tofu	4 Ounces	154	86

SUPPLEMENT FUNCTIONS

VITAMIN A
Aids in the treatment of many eye disorders; promotes bone growth, healthy hair, skin and teeth; helps protect mucous membranes and boosts resistance to respiratory and other infections; also fights acne.

VITAMIN B1 (THIAMIN)
Maintains muscle tissue and a healthy nervous system and heart; promotes growth; aids in digestion, particularly of carbohydrates.

VITAMIN B2 (RIBOFLAVIN)
Acts with other substances to utilize carbohydrates, fats and proteins; helps maintain mucous membranes and cell respiration; promotes good vision and healthy skin, hair and nails.

VITAMIN B3 (NIACIN)
Promotes a healthy nervous and digestive system; maintains healthy skin and hair; aids in circulation; assists in breakdown of carbohydrates, fats and proteins.

VITAMIN B5 (PANTOTHENIC ACID)
Aids cell building, healing and the formation and maintenance of adrenal hormones; helps in metabolism of carbohydrates, fats, and proteins.

VITAMIN B6 (PYRIDOXINE)
Aids in formation of red blood cells and metabolism of proteins and fats; helps regulate body fluids and nervous system; alleviates nausea.

SUPPLEMENT FUNCTIONS

VITAMIN B12 (COBALAMIN)
Forms and regulates red blood cells and helps prevent anemia; helps maintain a healthy nervous system; alleviates irritability and increases energy.

VITAMIN C (ASCORBIC ACID)
Aids production of collagen and red blood cells; maintains healthy blood vessels, bones, teeth and gums; helps body absorb iron; promotes healing.

VITAMIN D (CHOLECALCIFEROL)
Aids in formation and maintenance of bones and teeth; helps body absorb and utilize calcium and phosphorous; in adults it also helps maintain the nervous system, heart action, and blood clotting.

VITAMIN E (TOCOPHEROL)
Supplies oxygen to the body; aids in formation of red blood cells; helps maintain muscles and other tissues; protects Vitamin A and fatty acids from oxidation; promotes healing and is effective in preventing raised scar tissue.

VITAMIN K
Promotes proper blood clotting and helps prevent internal bleeding; aids normal liver functioning; enhances vitality.

BIOTIN
Aids in the formation of fatty acids; helps release energy from carbohydrates.

SUPPLEMENT FUNCTIONS

CALCIUM
Builds bones and teeth; maintains bone strength; eases muscle contraction; maintains cell membranes; aids in blood clotting, absorption of B12 and activation of enzymes.

CHLORINE (CHLORIDE)
Assists in the maintenance of the body's fluid and acid-base balance.

CHROMIUM
Assists in the metabolism of carbohydrates and fats.

COPPER
Assists in the formation of red blood cells; enhances iron absorption; stimulates healthy bones, blood vessels, nervous system functioning and the immune system.

FLUORINE (FLUORIDE)
Helps form bones and teeth.

FOLICIN (FOLIC ACID)
Aids in formation of red blood cells; helps maintain healthy nervous system; promotes mental health; essential for reproduction of all cells.

IODINE
Assists with cell metabolism and thyroid functioning.

IRON
Formation of hemoglobin in blood and myoglobin in muscles, which supply oxygen to cells; part of several enzymes and proteins.

SUPPLEMENT FUNCTIONS

L-CARNITINE
Helps with the production of energy through the transfer of long-chain fatty acids to the cells' mitochondria.

MAGNESIUM
Assists with bone formation and nerve and muscle functioning (including heart); helps to lessen depression and prevent calcium deposits, kidney stones and gallstones.

MANGANESE
Assists with metabolic functions; aids in bone growth and the function of nerves, bones and muscle.

PHOSPHORUS
Assists with energy production; helps build bones, teeth, cell membranes and genetic material.

POTASSIUM
Assists with development of muscles, nerve impulses, and heart and kidney functioning.

SELENIUM
Antioxidant, preventing breakdown of fats and other body chemicals; interacts with Vitamin E.

SODIUM
Helps regulate blood pressure and water balance in the body.

ZINC
Assists with enzyme activity related to cell division, growth and repair; aids with immune system functioning.

Knowing Your "Get Well" Choices

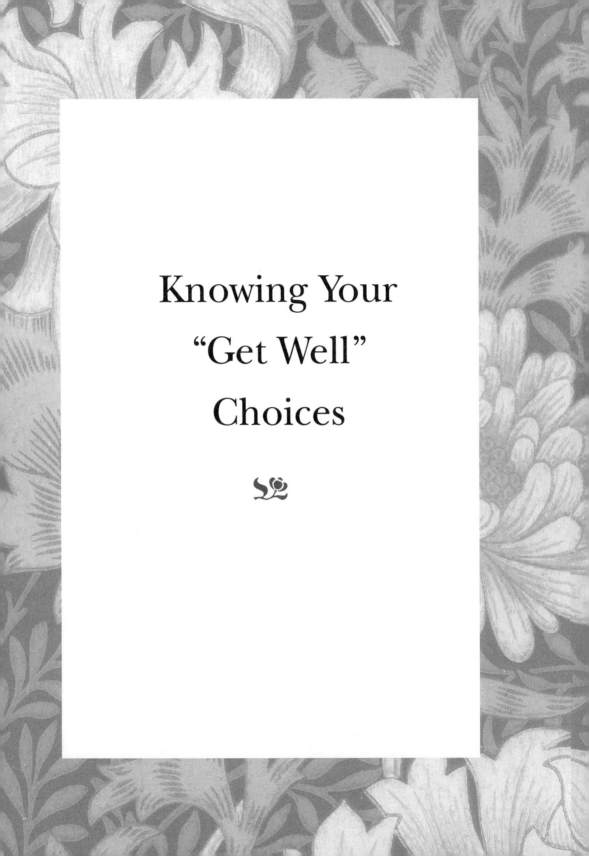

SYMPTOMS/CONCERNS	Standard Therapy	Herbal Remedies	Food	Supplements/Vitamins	Behaviour
Sleep Loss **Insomnia** **Sleep Disturbance** **Limits on Energy** **No Endurance** **Fatigue**	**Hormones** Estrogen, Progesterone: better sleep Testosterone: enhanced energy **Short-Term Sleep Remedies** Ambien Non-addictive sleep medication (Benadryl)	**For Sleep Loss/ Disturbance** Hops, Catnip Chamomile Ginseng Motherwort Chasteberry (Vitex) Passionflower St. John's Wort Valerian **For Tiredness** Oat straw Ginger Cayenne pepper Dandelion root Siberian ginseng Blessed thistle	**Avoid Excessive** Caffeine Chocolate Colas Alcohol Large evening meals **Consume** Frequent small meals Foods high in tryptophane, such as turkey **Drink** Warm nonfat milk before bedtime	**Try** Bioflavonoids Magnesium Potassium Vitamin B Complex Folic Acid **Anemia** Iron **Sleep Remedies** Melatonin Valerian **Homeopathic** Calm Forte Hylands	**Possible Causes** Decongestants Diet Pills Smoking **Try** AM daily exercise, meditation/Yoga, relaxation methods, relaxing activities, reading hot baths **Mental Health** Psychological Assessment and/ or Psychotherapy Psychiatric care and/or medication

SYMPTOMS/ CONCERNS	Standard Therapy	Herbal Remedies	Food	Supplements/ Vitamins	Behaviour
Heightened PMS Symptoms Tiredness Indifference Mood Swings Anxiety Irritability Depression Excessive Crying	**Hormone Therapy** Estrogen Testosterone **Mood-Enhancing Drugs** Prozac Zoloft Paxil **Anxiety** Progesterone (in some cases)	**For Anxiety** Valerian root Passionflower Peppermint Catnip Chamomile Hops **For Depression** St. John's Wort Oat straw Ginger Cayenne pepper Dandelion root Ginseng Blessed thistle **For PMS and Mood Swings** Chasteberry (Vitex) Chamomile	**For Mood Swings** Whole grains Liver Avoid Sugar **For PMS** Complex carbohydrates Tryptophanes Foods rich in Magnesium, Niacin and Vitamin B6 **For Calming Effect** Eggs, Turkey Soy products Dairy products **For Comfort** Pasta, Potatoes **Avoid Excessive** Alcohol, Caffeine Soft drinks with caffeine Junk foods	**For Anxiety and Irritability** Vitamin B Complex Vitamin B6 Bioflavonoids Melatonin Capsule **For Depression** Potassium Magnesium Vitamin B6 Vitamin B12 **For Mood Swings** Vitamin B Complex Vitamin B6 Vitamins C and E **For PMS** Calcium Magnesium Niacin Vitamin B6 Vitamin B Complex Vitamin C with Flax Oil Primrose Oil	**Meditation/ Relaxation Techniques** Yoga **Emotional Remedy** Psychological Assessment and/or Psychotherapy Psychiatric care and/or medication Daily Exercise

Symptoms/ Concerns	Standard Therapy	Herbal Remedies	Food	Supplements/ Vitamins	Behaviour
Breast Tenderness	**Hormone Therapy** Progesterone, Testosterone Prescription drugs Ibuprofen Aspirin Low-dose diuretics	**For Tenderness** Chasteberry (Vitex) **For Water Retention** Don quai root	**Avoid Excessive** Caffeine Fats Reduce salt intake	Calcium Vitamin B Complex Magnesium Vitamin E	Exercise 3-5 times per week
Mental Fuzziness Short Term Memory Loss Forgetfulness	**Hormone Therapy** Estrogen DHEA	Motherwort Valerian Passionflower Ginger Oat straw Cayenne pepper Dandelion root Siberian ginseng Blessed thistle	Eat small amounts frequently	**Increase Memory Performance** Gingko Tincture Gingko Gota Kola	**Increase Organization** Use notes, lists and reminders

282

Symptoms/Concerns	Standard Therapy	Herbal Remedies	Food	Supplements/Vitamins	Behaviour
Heavy Bleeding **Irregular Periods** **Spotting**	**For All Symptoms** **Progesterone** Low-dose birth control pills Have thyroid checked **If indicated** Surgical fibroid/polyp removal D & C Laser surgery to remove uterine lining Hysterectomy **For Cramps/Ovulatory Pain** Heat Ibuprofen Alleve	Red Clover Billberry **For Heavy Bleeding** Chasteberry (Vitex) Shepherds purse Blessed thistle Hawthorneberry Cherry, Grape skin Floradix Iron with herbs	**Avoid Excessive** Caffeine **Reduce** Animal fats in diet **Consume Foods with** Vitamin A, C, Iron and Bioflavonoids	**For Heavy Bleeding** Vitamin A Vitamin C Iron Bioflavonoids Calcium/Magnesium Essential fatty acids	Seek professional advice. Don't ignore symptoms. For heavy bleeding, rest and get tested for anemia.

SYMPTOMS/ CONCERNS	Standard Therapy	Herbal Remedies	Food	Supplements/ Vitamins	Behaviour
Headaches	**Hormone Therapy** Estrogen (if vascular)	Chamomile Catnip Chasteberry (Vitex) Peppermint Oil Feverfew Garden Sage Tea White Willow	**The Following Foods/Additives can trigger headaches** Aged cheese Aspartame Citrus fruit Chocolate Coffee Cured meats Eggplant Miso MSG Liver Peppers Potatoes Red wine Salt Sugar Tobacco Tomatoes Yogurt	Flax Liquid or Capsule Magnesium Niacin Primrose Oil Stress B Complex Vitamin B6 Vitamin C with Bioflavonoids	Exercise 3-5 times per week Meditation/ relaxation techniques Yoga **Emotional Remedy** Psychotherapy Psychiatric care and/or medication **Physical Causes** Allergies/infection Constipation Emotional stress Eye strain Food sensitivity Hypoglycemia Inflammation of nasal sinuses Muscle contraction of scalp/neck Systemic yeast disease

SYMPTOMS/ CONCERNS	Standard Therapy	Herbal Remedies	Food	Supplements/ Vitamins	Behaviour
Hot Flashes	**Hormone Therapy** Estrogen Progesterone **Non-Hormonal Medications** Clonidine Bellergal Aldomet Betablockers	**To Reduce the Frequency and Intensity** Black cohosh Sage Chasteberry (Vitex) Dandelion Yellow dock Milk Thistle Chickweed Elder Flower Oatstraw Motherwort Ginseng Blue Vervain Rosemary	**Avoid Excessive** Caffeine, Colas Chocolate Alcohol Spicy foods Sugar and sugar-rich foods (including fruit and fruit juices) Smoking Hot soups Hot drinks Large meals Fruits high in acid Ginger **Drink** Cold liquids **Eat Foods rich in** Vitamin B2, B6, B12 Vitamin C Vitamin E Bioflavonoids Hesperidin soy products	Bioflavonoids Hesperidin Vitamin B2, B6, B12 Vitamin C Vitamin E Calcium **Adrenal Support** Flax Oil Primrose Oil **Topical** Progesterone Cream	Daily Exercise Meditation and other relaxation techniques Yoga Slow, deep breathing Dress in layers Wear absorbent fabrics Carry a fan

Symptoms/ Concerns	Standard Therapy	Herbal Remedies	Food	Supplements/ Vitamins	Behaviour
Frequent Urination **Vaginal Yeast Conditions** **Bladder/ Urinary Tract Infections**	Estrogen Empty bladder frequently Kegel exercises and behavior modification; in rare cases, surgery **Yeast Conditions** Anti-fungal vaginal inserts or oral medications: Yeast Guard Vagisil Yeast Control Gyne-Lotrimin Mycelex-7 Monistat-7 Diflucan 1 oral tablet = 7-day treatment **Bacterial Infections** Antibiotics	**For Frequent Urination** Chasteberry (Vitex) **For Infections** Goldenseal Uva ursi Blackberry root Wintergreen	**Avoid the Following Bladder Irritants** Artificial sweeteners Black tea White sugar Citrus fruit juices Tomatoes Iced drinks Pineapples Carbonated drinks Spicy foods Chocolate Acid-forming foods Concentrated starches e.g. yams, potatoes Fried and fatty foods Foods with yeast **Consume** 4 oz. glass of water every 1/2 hour Cranberry juice (unsweetened) Yogurt	**Consume** Yogurt Foods that are rich in Vitamin A, B, C, E and Zinc Add flax seed oil to diet Acidophilis Beta Carotene and/or Vitamin A Buffered Vitamin C Garlic Green Algae products Plant Enzyme/ Protease or Bromeline Carrot Beef Cucumber Juice Parsley Freeze-dried cranberry capsules	**Take Care of Yourself** Eat a balanced diet Get plenty of rest Reduce stress Yeast-free diet Kegel exercises Relax while urinating Urinate after sex

SYMPTOMS/ CONCERNS	Standard Therapy	Herbal Remedies	Food	Supplements/ Vitamins	Behaviour
Vaginal Dryness and/or Itching	**Hormone Therapy** Estrogen replacement Vaginal estrogen creams, gels, and suppositories **Non-hormonal lubricants** Vagisil Lubrin Feminease Replens Gyne Moistrin	Don quai root Acidophilus capsules inserted vaginally Wild yam root ointment	**Consume** Essential fatty acids (EFAs) **Avoid Excessive** Caffeine Alcohol Sugar	**Applied topically** Calendula cream **Chew** Don quai root **Inserted vaginally** Vitamin A vaginal suppositories	**Explore causes** Antihistamines and other drugs that have drying characteristics **Avoid** Douching Deodorant tampons Scented bath oils, salts or soaps Pantyliners with deodorant Pantyhose Panties with synthetic fibers

287

SYMPTOMS/ CONCERNS	Standard Therapy	Herbal Remedies	Food	Supplements/ Vitamins	Behaviour
Uncomfortable Intercourse	**Hormone Therapy** Estrogen Testosterone Low-dose, topically applied, resinbased estrogen **Non-Hormonal Vaginal Moisturizers** Replens Gyne-Moistrin Sexual Lubricants (water-based) Astroglide Ortho Personal Lube Lubrin	Chasteberry (Vitex) Don quai root Acidophilus capsules inserted vaginally Wild yam root ointment	**Avoid Excessive** Sugar Caffeine Alcohol Fried foods Processed foods **For Vaginal Lubrication, Consume** Essential fatty acids (EFAs) Foods rich in Zinc and Vitamins B, C, and E	Zinc Vitamin E Vitamin B Vitamin C Niacin Copper Iodine Magnesium Calcium Flax Oil Primrose Oil	**Exercise/Relaxation** Engage in exercises that help you feel fit, physical and sexy Yoga Kegel exercises **Emotional** Psychological Assessment and/or Psychotherapy **Sexual Health** Sexual intercourse or masturbation with orgasm weekly Read books or view videos on the subject

SYMPTOMS/ CONCERNS	Standard Therapy	Herbal Remedies	Food	Supplements/ Vitamins	Behaviour
Gastric Upset Constipation Flatulence/ Gas	**Medical Exam and Diagnosis** To rule out ulcer or check for any serious condition **Medications and Suggestions** Estrogen replacement Change in diet Antacids Laxatives	**For Gastric Upset** Chamomile Peppermint Aloe Vera Licorice Root Slippery Elm Flax Seed Bitter Herbs **For Constipation** Psyllium Seeds Ginger tea	**To Relieve Gastric Upset and Constipation** Fiber-rich foods 3-4 prunes before bedtime Applesauce Yogurt Soups, liquids and other soft foods Papaya Cooked greens **Avoid Excessive** White flour products Meat **Drink** Electrolyte drink w/ no sugar I-modium Miso broth **Flatulence/Gas** Avoid foods that give you problems	**Gastric Upset** Acidophilus capsules **Flatulence/Gas** Acidophilus capsules Charcoal tablets Plant/Pancreatic enzymes Beano Lactaid Simethicone products (Gas-X, Phazyme, Mylicon) **Constipation** Acidophilus capsules Aloe vera juice Fiber supplements	**Gastric Upset/Gas** Check whether you're gulping air while eating Don't eat too fast Notice if you have irregular breathing or have a tendency to swallow air during tasks or talking **For constipation** Increase activity Drink 6-8 glasses of water daily

289

Symptoms/ Concerns	Standard Therapy	Herbal Remedies	Food	Supplements/ Vitamins	Behaviour
Joint and Muscle Aches/Pain **Limited Range of Motion**	**For Inflammation** Advil Motrin Aspirin Alleve **For Arthritic Pain** Consult with your physician Estrogen replacement or as advised dhea	**Herbal Teas** Burdock Black cohosh Blue cohosh Nettles Valerian root **For Joint Pain** Cleavers	Essential fatty acids (EFAs) High fiber **Avoid** Acid-forming foods Alcohol Meat Sugar **Consume** Night shade family foods, tomatoes, bell peppers, potatoes, eggplant	Vitamin E Glycocamine Sulfate Niacin/Niacinamine Shark Cartilage **Topically** Arnica Oil or Lotion Tiger Balm Traumel Cream Ben Gay Aspercream	Massage Whirlpool/Jacuzzi Daily Exercise, swimming especially soothing Yoga

SYMPTOMS/CONCERNS	Standard Therapy	Herbal Remedies	Food	Supplements/Vitamins	Behaviour
Skin Problems: Acne Sensitivity Wrinkles Discoloration Rashes Bruising	Retin-A Renova Prescription Strength Glycolic Acid Acutane Deep skin peels	Chasteberry (Vitex) Chaste tree	**Avoid Excessive** Caffeine Cola Diet drinks Alcohol Excess oil Saturated fats Hydrogenated spreads Sugar Refined/enriched flours and grains	Vitamin A Vitamin E Vitamin B Complex Vitamin B6 Niacin Vitamin C Iodine Zinc Iron Calcium	Meditation Exercise 3-5 times per week Yoga **To Protect the Skin** Stop smoking Use sun screen, at least 15 SPF Large hats
Unwanted Hair Growth on Face and Chest	**Hormone Therapy** Estrogen Anti-testosterone medication Rule out hypothyroidism	Chasteberry (Vitex)	**Consume** High-quality protein Complex carbohydrates Vegetables Whole grains Fruit Calcium-rich foods		**For Unwanted Hair Growth** Bleaching Hair Removal Creams Electrolysis Waxing

SYMPTOMS/ CONCERNS	Standard Therapy	Herbal Remedies	Food	Supplements/ Vitamins	Behaviour
Breast Disease	**Medical** Regular medical check-ups Mammograms Biopsy **For Breast Cancer** Chemotherapy Mastectomy Lumpectomy Radiation Hormone manipulation therapy	Alfalfa Kelp	**Avoid Excessive** Caffeine Carbonated soft drinks Chocolate Cocoa Reduce fat intake Meat intake Consume daily variety of fruits and vegetables Low-fat diet High-fiber diet Nutrient-rich foods **Add Foods with** Vitamins C, E, A (beta carotene) and selenium	**For Fibrocystic Breast Disease** Vitamin A Vitamin E Iodine Selenium **For Breast Cancer** Iodine Selenium Vitamin A Vitamin C	Breast self-examination Maintain a desirable body weight Exercise 3-5 times per week Meditation and other relaxation techniques Yoga **Emotional** Psychological Assessment and/or Psychotherapy Psychiatric care and /or medication
Skin Cancer	Regular medical check-ups and screening tests Biopsy				

SYMPTOMS/CONCERNS	Standard Therapy	Herbal Remedies	Food	Supplements/Vitamins	Behaviour
Thyroid Problems	**Low** Thyroid replacement therapy Estrogen replacement **High** Anti-thyroid medicines Radioactive Iodine	Bay Berry Bark Dulse Gota Kola Irish Moss Kelp Rhubarb Root Sarsaparilla	**Avoid Excessive** Brussels sprouts Cabbage Caffeine **Consume** 75% fresh foods Iodine-rich foods Vitamin A-rich foods	**For Hypothyroid** Vitamin C Vitamin E Iodine Primrose Oil Selenium Calcium/ Magnesium/ Potassium capsules Emulsified A or Beta Carotene Raw Thyroid Raw Pituitary Raw Adrenal substance Thyroid Glandular w/ Tyrosine	Exercise 3-5 times per week Meditation/relaxation techniques Yoga **Emotional** Psychological Assessment and/or Psychotherapy Psychiatric care and/or medication **Avoid** Fluorescent lights Smoking
Sub-clinical Hypo/Hyper					
Hypo(low)					
Hyper(high)					

293

Symptoms/Concerns	Standard Therapy	Herbal Remedies	Food	Supplements/Vitamins	Behaviour
Colon Cancer	Early diagnosis through screening tests **Medical treatment** Radiation Chemotherapy Immunologic agents Surgery		**Avoid Excessive** Alcohol Caffeine **Consume** A lowfat/high-fiber diet Fruits and vegetables (daily) Foods high in Vitamin A **Reduce** Fat intake Salt-cured, smoked and nitrate pre-served foods Meat intake	Vitamin A Antioxidants Beta Carotene Selenium Vitamin E Vitamin B12 Folic Acid Zinc Germanium Acidophilus Fiber Products Chlorophyll Garlic	Maintain a desirable body weight Exercise 3-5 times per week Meditation and other relaxation techniques Yoga Enemas, if advised **Emotional** Psychological Assessment and/or Psychotherapy Psychiatric care and/or medication

SYMPTOMS/ CONCERNS	Standard Therapy	Herbal Remedies	Food	Supplements/ Vitamins	Behaviour
Heart Disease **Heart Attack** **Stroke** **Hypertension** **Other Cardio-vascular Problems**	**Prevention** Exercise and healthy diet **Hormone Therapy** Estrogen **Over-the-Counter Drugs** Baby aspirin **With Disease** Medications and possibly surgery	Peppermint Yellow dock Uva ursi Parsley Alfalfa Raspberry leaves Nettles Dandelion greens Violet leaves Lamb's quarters Sage Chickweed Horsetail Black cohosh Rosehips	**Avoid Excessive** Alcohol Caffeine Salt Processed meats high in fat, salt and preservatives **Reduce** Fat intake Cholesterol **Consume** Lowfat diet High-fiber diet Foods high in Vitamin A, C, E and Calcium Foods high in soluble fiber Small meals	**For Cerebral Artery Disease** Manganese **For Coronary Artery Disease** Magnesium **For Hypertension** Potassium Calcium Vitamin E **For Heart Disease** Potassium **For Cardiovascular Health** Vitamin C Vitamin E	Maintain desirable body weight Avoid smoking Aerobic exercise 3-5 times per week Meditation and other relaxation techniques Yoga **Emotional** Psychological Assessment and/or Psychotherapy Psychiatric care and/or medica-tion

SYMPTOMS/ CONCERNS	Standard Therapy	Herbal Remedies	Food	Supplements/ Vitamins	Behaviour
Osteoporosis	**Hormone Therapy** Estrogen Testosterone Non-Hormonal Medication Alendronate Etidronate Calcitonin	Red raspberry leaf Comfrey Oatstraw Kelp Nettles Horsetail Sage	**Avoid Excessive** Alcohol Caffeine Carbonated beverages Excess protein Salt Saturated fats Smoking Sugar **Consume** A low-protein/low-fat/low-salt diet Adequate dairy products Foods high in calcium Sea vegetables **Reduce** Red meat intake Foods high in phosphorus	Malic Acid Boric Acid Manganese Magnesium Silicon Copper Zinc Folic Acid Boron Calcium Vitamin D Floradix Iron with herbs HCL (High potency digestive enzymes)	Weight-bearing exercise 3 hours per week Aerobic exercise 3 hours per week Yoga Get sun exposure (with sunscreen protection) Avoid uncoated aluminum pots and pans

Symptoms/ Concerns	Standard Therapy	Herbal Remedies	Food	Supplements/ Vitamins	Behaviour
Uterine Fibroids **Ovarian Cysts**	Consult with your physician Check for underlying hormonal imbalance		**Avoid Excessive** Dairy products **Consume** Foods rich in Vitamin A, C, B6 and Folic Acid	Vitamin A Folic Acid Vitamin B6 Vitamin C w/ Bioflavonoids Vitamin E	Exercise 3-5 times per week

Your Health Advisor and You

Peter P. Farmer, M.D.   Kathy Farmer, P.A.

❧

Are you 100 percent satisfied with your visit to your doctor? You can be, if you decide that you have something to do with how satisfied you are, and prepare yourself ahead of time by answering the following five questions:

- Why are you seeing this particular doctor?
- What do you want to be sure to say?
- What's possible from your relationship with this doctor?
- What specific outcomes do you intend to produce with this doctor?
- (At the end of your visit) Are you satisfied with your visit?

Often we read information from the point of view of whether we agree or disagree with the information presented. These thoughts and recommendations are not offered as the truth and are therefore best read by asking "what new way of approaching my health might be available here?" Rather than as a formula, this is intended as a format to stimulate your thinking. The questions are applicable each time you see a doctor. The answers you get will be valuable because they will be YOUR answers in YOUR life. Take on one or two questions. Over time you will cover the whole list and add your own questions.

WHY ARE YOU SEEING THIS PARTICULAR DOCTOR?

1. Have you seen this doctor before?
2. Who referred you to this doctor?

3. What have you heard from friends or other healthcare providers about this doctor?

4. Is this the right doctor for the condition you have?

   The previous questions have more to do with the qualities of the doctor. The following questions in this section have more to do with you and require introspection on your part.

5. Do you trust this doctor? If you don't, why not? If the reason is resolvable or obviously not related to this doctor (e.g. he reminds you of your Uncle Ed who's a drunk), then do what you need to do to re-establish the trust. If the reason is not resolvable, find a new doctor.

6. Who will be responsible and accountable for your health? You? Your doctor? The answer to this can vary with each situation.

7. How much authority do you want to give your doctor? A possible goal: being an active and informed patient who makes decisions in partnership with your doctor.

WHAT DO YOU WANT TO BE SURE TO SAY?

1. Do you speak the same language as your doctor or do you need an interpreter?

2. What happened? Include whatever you think (or suspect) is important. For example: When did your symptoms start? How would you characterize your discomfort? Is there any association between your symptoms and what do you do? What makes your symptoms better or worse?

3. What can you anticipate your doctor asking? For example: Do you have any allergies? What treatments have you done or had? Have you followed the previous treatment plan, taken your prescriptions, etc.? What significant past history do you have? What is your family and social history including contacts with similar symptoms?

4. What do you want to bring with you in order to supply necessary information? For example: medications including vitamins, herbs, and supplements. How you are currently taking them? What insurance cards, HMO Plan Physician Rosters, or payment information do you need? Do you have a record of your prior surgeries, illnesses, and injuries? Do

you have a summary sheet of your medical problems and their current status?

5. What specific questions and concerns do you have? Include the seemingly silly questions. Write them down, listing the most important first. For example: When I stand up the room spins. Does this mean I'm having a stroke?

6. What reading could you do to clarify your questions? You may include searching the Internet regarding your particular problem.

7. What expectations or requests do you have? For example, do you expect to have this problem resolved or to receive specific answers on this visit? Ask specific questions so you can get specific answers and a better understanding.

8. Are you being open and honest about your smoking, drug, alcohol, and sexual practices? Your doctor cannot put the pieces together to get answers for you if some of the pieces are missing.

9. Have you informed the doctor about previous treatments? Are you concerned he or she won't agree? Were previous treatments unpleasant? How does the current recommendation relate to your past experience? For example, you had sever pain from a cortisone injection and are afraid that your doctor will recommend the same treatment.

WHAT'S POSSIBLE FROM YOUR RELATIONSHIP WITH THIS DOCTOR?

It is possible to take on achieving a state of health unpredictable from your current health conditions or disabilities and still be appropriate to them. If you are actively engaged in being as healthy as possible, the following questions will be valuable.

1. What actions taken now will give you the kind of health required to do what you want to be doing in five, ten, twenty-five, or fifty years?

2. What habits or practices do you want to alter or institute now?

3. What could you take on now that would be healthy, fun, and satisfying? For example: 50 percent of the factors affecting your health are related to your lifestyle and are therefore already in your control.

It is also possible to take on establishing an extraordinary relationship with your doctor. If you see this could make a difference for you, consider the following approach:

1. Assume your doctor is interested in you and what you have to say, no matter how busy he or she seems.
2. Remember that doctors are human beings with individual lives and personalities and whether you were satisfied or dissatisfied with any previous doctor or visit has nothing to do with this doctor or this visit.
3. A challenging, confronting relationship is usually unproductive and dissatisfying for both the patient and the doctor.
4. How can you empower your doctor to be his or her best? Can your doctor be for you just like Hawkeye Pierce, Marcus Welby, or your favorite hero from "E.R." or "Chicago Hope"?

WHAT SPECIFIC OUTCOMES DO YOU INTEND TO PRODUCE FROM THIS VISIT?

1. What can happen during this visit that will make a significant difference in your health?
2. Are the outcomes you want to produce written down?
3. Do you have sufficient time scheduled to accomplish what you intend? For example: a complete history and physical evaluation requires more than a fifteen-minute appointment.
4. Are your intended outcomes realistic and reasonable? Medical practice is more an art than a perfect science. If you stop crediting it with more certainty and curing power than it has and begin relating to it as it is, you will be more effective and satisfied.
5. Your doctor will develop a plan for further investigation or treatment.
   a) Do you understand the plan? What's the timeline?
   b) What difficulties or discomforts can you expect following the plan?
   c) Do you agree with the plan? Tell the truth about what you are going to do and what you are not going to do.
   d) Is there reading material your doctor can recommend regarding your symptoms, disease, or treatment plan?
   e) Ask your doctor about prescribed medication:

What is the name of the drug and what is it supposed to do? How and when should you take it and for how long? What food, drinks, and other medicines or activities should be avoided while taking this drug? Are there any side effects and what do I do if they occur? Do you have any written information available about this drug?

6. Who should you speak to if you have questions after you leave? If questions arise, call back.

ARE YOU SATISFIED WITH YOUR VISIT?

If your answer is yes, congratulations! If you are dissatisfied, say so. Does your dissatisfaction have to do with a broken agreement? Ask yourself the following questions regarding broken agreements and communicate the answers:

1. What agreement was broken? Problems often arise because an agreement regarding something to be done is assumed. If you expected your doctor to do something but never made the request, make the request now.

2. How was the agreement broken? Did your doctor not call back when a call was promised? Did you fail to take your medication as it was prescribed?

3. What new request that will resolve your dissatisfaction can you make? If you are unable to resolve your dissatisfaction, go to another doctor.

In conclusion, getting the most out of your relationship with your doctor requires preparation, open and honest communication, and taking on being responsible for your own health. Establish a strong relationship with your doctor. Think about what might be possible out of your visit. Know specifically what you want to accomplish. This will give you a much greater chance of reaching your goal. Working with these questions over time will assist you in having an unpredictable relationship with your doctor that could open the door to an extraordinary state of health.

DIAGNOSTIC QUESTIONNAIRE:
YOUR HEALTH HISTORY IS YOU

This comprehensive survey was developed by John C. Arpels, M.D., for his San Francisco Gynecology & Menopausal Medicine practice. Use it to learn about your own health picture and to share with your health advisor.

Name _____

What age are you? _____

Are you allergic to any medicine(s)?   no   yes

Identify _____

_____

What medicine(s) do you take? _____

_____

Have you ever been diagnosed with cancer?   no   yes

What type and date _____

Have you ever had an operation?   no   yes

Type and date _____

Have you ever been hospitalized?   no   yes

Reason and date _____

Have you been seriously injured?   no   yes

Type(s) and date _____

Have you ever had a pelvic infection

(uterus, tubes, ovaries, etc.)?   no   yes

What kind(s) and date?_____

How often do you have periods? _____

Date of last normal one _____

Date of period before last one _____

Have they become less regular?   no   yes

Have they become more frequent?   no   yes

Have they become less frequent?   no   yes

Do you have cramps with your periods?   no   yes

Is the total amount of blood flow or frequency

of periods different now?   no   yes

If so, how? _____

Did/Do any of the following apply to you?

- periods beginning before age twelve   no   yes

- light menstrual flow during age twenty-forty years   no   yes

- forty-five or more days between periods
    when twenty to forty years   no   yes

- loss of periods from stress or exercise   no   yes

If menopausal, when was your last period? _____

At what age did your mother become menopausal? _____

Older sister's menopause _____

If you've had children, did you experience
    post-delivery blues?   no   yes

Did/Do you have bothersome PMS symptoms
    or monthly mood swings?   no   yes

If "yes," describe _____

Do you routinely use a diuretic or laxative?   no   yes

If so, please name _____

Do you have a high stress job or lifestyle?   no   yes

Do you smoke cigarettes now?   no   yes

If so, daily use _____

Have you smoked in the past?   no   yes

If so, how long and daily use _____

Please indicate how any of the following symptoms apply to you currently, using the following categories:

none — no noticeable symptoms.

mild — symptoms are hardly noticeable; no treatment necessary.

moderate — symptoms are noticeable; not incapacitating; possibly require some treatment, medication or behavior adjustments.

severe — incapacitating; treatment, medication or therapy is needed to function/relieve pain.

Decreased short-term memory? none   mild   moderate   severe

Difficulty solving problems?   none   mild   moderate   severe

Increased forgetfulness?   none   mild   moderate   severe

Slower thinking?   none   mild   moderate   severe

Decreased ability to do multiple tasks?

                          none   mild   moderate   severe

Decreased mental energy?   none   mild   moderate   severe

Inappropriate moodiness?   none   mild   moderate   severe

Inappropriate depression?   none   mild   moderate   severe

Excessive crying?   none   mild   moderate   severe

Misplaced anger?   none   mild   moderate   severe

Inappropriate irritability?   none   mild   moderate   severe

Excessive anxiety?   none   mild   moderate   severe

Increased nervousness?   none   mild   moderate   severe

Decreased tolerance?	none	mild	moderate	severe
Reduced sense of well-being?	none	mild	moderate	severe
Loss of usual interest in things?	none	mild	moderate	severe
Loss of focus?	none	mild	moderate	severe

Panic attacks or fear of leaving home?

	none	mild	moderate	severe
Any claustrophobia?	none	mild	moderate	severe
Worry about aging?	none	mild	moderate	severe
Loss of appetite?	none	mild	moderate	severe
Thoughts of suicide?	none	mild	moderate	severe

᭛

Daytime hot flashes or flushing?

	none	mild	moderate	severe

Nighttime hot flashes or hotness?

	none	mild	moderate	severe
Nighttime sweating?	none	mild	moderate	severe

Heat intolerance/cold intolerance?

	none	mild	moderate	severe
Difficulty getting to sleep?	none	mild	moderate	severe
Increased interrupted sleep?	none	mild	moderate	severe
Increased tiredness	none	mild	moderate	severe

History of headaches?	none	mild	moderate	severe
More frequent headaches?	none	mild	moderate	severe
Increased joint pain?	none	mild	moderate	severe
Increased muscle aches?	none	mild	moderate	severe
Drier eyes?	none	mild	moderate	severe
Decrease in visual clarity?	none	mild	moderate	severe
Drier skin?	none	mild	moderate	severe
Increased bruising?	none	mild	moderate	severe

Unusual skin tingling or burning?

	none	mild	moderate	severe
More brittle hair or hair loss?	none	mild	moderate	severe
Deterioration of fingernails?	none	mild	moderate	severe
Drier mouth?	none	mild	moderate	severe
Increased heartburn?	none	mild	moderate	severe
More indigestion?	none	mild	moderate	severe
Chest feels full or painful?	none	mild	moderate	severe

Heart palpitations or irregularity?

	none	mild	moderate	severe
Ringing in the ears?	none	mild	moderate	severe

Increased dizziness or loss of balance?

	none	mild	moderate	severe

Acne?   none   mild   moderate   severe

Increased dental or gum problems?

                                    none   mild   moderate   severe

❧

Increased loss of urine?   none   mild   moderate   severe

More frequent urination?   none   mild   moderate   severe

More bladder infections?   none   mild   moderate   severe

❧

Decrease in vaginal lubrication?

                                    none   mild   moderate   severe

Discomfort during sexual intercourse?

                                    none   mild   moderate   severe

Longer time to orgasm?   none   mild   moderate   severe

Painful orgasm?   none   mild   moderate   severe

Increase in vaginal infections?   none   mild   moderate   severe

Decrease in sexual desire?   none   mild   moderate   severe

Burning or pain in skin of vulva?

                                    none   mild   moderate   severe

Decrease in sexual fantasy?   none   mild   moderate   severe

❧

Are you bothered by any other symptoms which you feel might be related to your hormone changes, menopause or midlife?

no   yes

Describe _____

Is there a history of the following cancer(s) in your family?
If yes, identify family member(s).

Breast   no   yes

Colon   no   yes

Ovarian   no   yes

Uterine   no   yes

Prostate   no   yes

Is there any other form of cancer in your family?   no   yes

What kind(s)? _____

Is there a history of osteoporosis or hip fractures in your family?

no   yes

Please identify _____

Do you actively engage in some form of exercise at least twice a week?   no   yes

What type?_____

Have you ever had a bone density scan?   no   yes

What kind? _____

Date of last one _____

Have you ever had an abnormal PAP smear?   no   yes

What year?_____

Date of last normal PAP _____

Have you ever had a mammogram?   no   yes

Date of most recent _____

Results _____

Have you ever had a sigmoidoscopy or colonoscopy?

                                                      no   yes

Date of most recent _____

Results _____

Is there a history of cardiovascular disease in your family?

                                                      no   yes

High blood pressure?   no   yes

Please identify _____

Heart disease?   no   yes

Please identify _____

Stroke?   no   yes

Please identify _____

High cholesterol? no yes

Please identify _____

What is your total cholesterol level? _____

Date last tested _____

What is your HDL ratio to total cholesterol? _____

Date last tested _____

What is your blood pressure level? _____

Date last tested _____

What is your current weight and height? _____

Do you consider yourself twenty pounds over your desired weight?

no yes

What is your lean body mass to fat ratio?

Do you take Vitamin A, C, or E on a regular basis?

no yes

Is your daily diet high in fruits/vegetables? no yes

Do you drink more than two cups/glasses of caffeine-containing
beverages per day (coffee, tea, cola, etc.)? no yes

Identify _____

Is your diet high in daily calcium (dairy products, broccoli, greens,
beans, soy products, etc.)? no yes

Do you take a calcium supplement? no yes

Type and dosage _____

Do you consume more than six glasses of alcoholic
   beverage(s) per week?   no   yes

Identify _____

Is your diet high in fiber?   no   yes

Is your diet high in fats (oil, cheese, beef, nuts, avocado, etc.)?

                                      no   yes

Is your diet high in cholesterol (dairy products shell
   fish, pork, sausage, lunch meats)?   no   yes

Has your thyroid function been tested?   no   yes

Date _____

Was it normal? _____

Has your glucose (sugar) level been tested?   no   yes

Date _____

Are there any significant medical problems in your family
   that have not already been identified?   no   yes

Is there a history of Dementia or Alzheimer's in
   you family?   no   yes

If yes, whom? _____

What type? _____

Is there any additional information that you feel
   might be helpful?   no   yes

If so, please describe: _____

10 Dangerous Drug Combinations

These pairs of drugs can have dangerous, even fatal effects. If you are using any of these combinations, contact your physician for alternatives.

Seldane— Erythromycin

Mevacor— Lopid

Coumadin— Tagamet

Calan— Duraquin

Theo-Dur— Tagamet

Lanoxin (Digoxin)— Calan

Prozac— Dilantin

Halcion— Erythromycin

Eldepryl— Norpramine

Tagamet— Dilantin

Source: *Worst Pills/Best Pills News*. Adapted by Emily K. Wolman.

GLOSSARY

acne — skin eruptions; often take the form of rosacea or contact dermatitis in midlife women

allergies — abnormal hypersensitivity to substances that are ordinarily harmless; common allergies affect the respiratory passages and skin, although they may also affect the digestive tract, joints, kidneys, and nervous system; can be acquired with age and are sometimes associated with such emotional upsets as anxiety, fear, and strong excitement

amenorrhea — when menstrual periods stop and the cause is not related to menopause

androgens — hormones with male-like characteristics, e.g. testosterone

anemia — below-normal amount of red blood cells due to poor diet, excessive uterine bleeding, and other causes; iron supplements may be prescribed if blood test indicates; symptoms: loss of energy, pounding heart, breath shortness

antidepressants — medications used to treat depressive illness

arteries — the vessels that carry blood from the heart to the rest of the body

arthritis — inflammation of joint(s)

asthma — a condition marked by recurrent attacks of wheezing and labored breathing due to spasmodic constriction of the bronchial area; as with allergies, asthma can be developed in midlife, sometimes as a result of allergies themselves; can also be due to recurrent bronchial and/or sinus infections

atherosclerosis — hardening of the arteries

Bartholin's glands — two glands on each side of the vaginal opening that secrete mucus

basal body temperature — an oral, rectal, or basal mercury thermometer is placed in the armpit for ten minutes before rising in the morning; readings below 97.8 degrees may indicate low thyroid; women still menstruating should test on second and third day of period; no alcohol should be drunk the night before

bladder—a membranous sac in which urine is stored before it is released

blood clot—a jelly-like substance over the ends and inside of a blood vessel

breakthrough bleeding—vaginal bleeding that can occur while taking female hormones or oral contraceptives, or from other causes that should be diagnosed

calories—a measure of heat units used to determine how much energy is present in the food one consumes

cancer—uncontrolled growth of abnormal cells that destroy healthy cells

cardiovascular—refers to the heart and blood vessels

chronic dermatitis—inflammation of the skin with symptoms including itching, crustiness, blisters, redness, watery discharges, or other changes in normal skin

cervix—the lower end of the uterus between the uterus and the vagina

cholesterol—an essential steroid chemical; excess implicated in heart disease

chronic—present or developing over a long period of time; opposite of acute

chronic fatigue syndrome (CFS)—an illness characterized by fever, achy muscles, severe drowsiness, and tiredness that can last for several months or longer; difficult to diagnose

climacteric—designates a woman's transition from her child-bearing years to her non-childbearing life and a period of time after, covering ages thirty-five to sixty-five; late climacteric—the years after menstruation ceases, between fifty-five and sixty-five

congenital—present at and existing since birth, but not inherited

contact dermatitis—skin condition marked by swelling, itching, oozing, or blistering; usually caused by direct contact with a substance to which the person is sensitive or allergic; is an affliction that occurs in midlife for many women

coronary artery disease—fatty disease of the arteries of the heart that can lead to blood clotting

D & C—a common gynecologic procedure in which the cervix is opened or stretched (dilation) and the inner surface is cleansed with an instrument called a curette

DHEA-sulfate—an abundant hormone secreted by the adrenal glands that declines with aging; appears in supplementation therapy to have some protective influences for certain diseases, joint pain, mood balancing, memory, energy, libido, menopause symptoms, and the immune system

diabetes—deficiency disease due to lack of insulin; Adult Type II requires a specific diet, exercise, and sometimes oral medications as treatment rather than insulin shots as in Type I diabetes; occurs in midlife women, most often those with excess body fat, and more frequently after menopause

diuretic—a medication or liquid such as coffee, tea, or water that promotes urine secretion

dosage—the strength and frequency at which a drug should be taken

dysmenorrhea—pain and/or cramps during menstrual period, sometimes accompanied by headaches, fatigue, irritability, and mental depression

edema—abnormal accumulation of fluid in the body that causes swelling

endocrinologist—a physician specializing in the diagnosis and treatment of glandular disorders

endometriosis—condition in which fragments of the uterine lining implant themselves in other parts of (or on organs within) the pelvic cavity, e.g. ovaries, fallopian tubes; diagnosed by laparoscopy

ERT—estrogen replacement therapy

estrogen—the female sex hormone produced by the ovaries

fallopian tube—the tube from the uterus that opens near the ovary and acts as a duct for the sperm and egg fibroid tumors—benign fiber and muscle tumor(s) that may cause heavy or abnormal bleeding; there are three growth patterns: within the uterine walls (most common), on the outer walls of the uterus, or under the uterine lining and inside the uterine cavity

follicle—a sac containing an egg and fluid in the ovary

FSH (follicle-stimulating hormone)—the pituitary sex hormone that signals the ovaries to release an egg each month

gland—body structure that secretes chemicals or fluids

hormones—chemical substances that act as messengers; mainly produced by the endocrine glands, they travel through the bloodstream to the cells and organs where they perform a specific regulatory effect, e.g., insulin, estrogen, progesterone

HRT—hormone replacement therapy, similar to ERT but includes estrogen plus progestin/progesterone treatment

hypothalamus—the coordinating center of the brain that lies beneath the thalamus gland and above the pituitary gland

hysterectomy—surgical removal of the uterus

insomnia—an abnormal wakefulness that inhibits the ability to fall asleep easily or to remain asleep throughout the night

luteinizing hormone (LH)—the pituitary hormone that stimulates release of the egg from the graafian follicle

kidney disease (nephritis)—inflammation of the kidney; destructive disease that may involve and damage the internal membranes

libido—sexual desire and drive

menarche—the first menstrual period

"natural" estrogens—pharmaceutical production of estrogens for estrogen replacement therapy (ERT), mirroring on a molecular level those naturally produced by the body

oophorectomy—surgical removal of one or both ovaries

ovaries—the female organs that contain eggs and make sex hormones

ovulation—release of the egg from the follicle of the ovary

PAP smear—scraping from the cervix to detect abnormal changes and cancerous conditions

pelvis—bony basin around the lower abdominal organs

peri-menopause—the years just before and after menstruation ceases, between forty-five and fifty-five

progesterone—an essential female sex hormone that promotes healthy functioning of the female reproductive system

progestin—medication formulated to act like the female hormone progesterone for hormone replacement therapy; e.g. norethindrone

progestogen—see progestin; e.g. Provera®

prolapse—dropping or sagging of the uterus, vagina, and bladder due to loss of pelvic support

psychogenic—that which is caused by an emotional or psychological problem

rosacea—a chronic skin condition that affects the forehead, cheeks, and nose with flushing, followed by red coloration and acne-like lesions; not uncommon at midlife for women

renal failure—kidney failure

reproductive organs—ovaries, fallopian tubes, uterus, and vagina

somatic—pertaining to the body

spotting—irregular, slight vaginal bleeding between periods

stress incontinence—inability to hold urine properly during coughing, laughing, sneezing, or exercise

subcutaneous—under the skin

surgical menopause—menopause following surgical removal of the ovaries

symptom—the feeling that alerts the body that something is wrong

syndrome—a set of symptoms that cluster as a group

testosterone—the hormone made by the testes, the ovaries and the adrenal glands

tranquilizers—medications to reduce anxiety

transdermal — through the skin

urethra — the tube from the bladder through which urine is discharged from the body

vagina — muscular canal leading from the external genitalia to the uterus

vaginal smear — scraping of the vaginal wall for laboratory testing

varicose veins — swollen, distended veins, especially of the legs

veins — the vessels that carry blood from the body to the heart

vulva — external female genitalia

RESOURCES AND PROFESSIONAL ORGANIZATIONS

Alliance for Aging Research 2021 K Street NW, Suite 305, Washington, DC 20006 (202) 293-2856.

Alzheimer's Disease Education and Referral Center P.O. Box 8250, Silver Springs, MD 20907-8250 (301) 495-3311.

American Academy of Dermatology 930 N. Meacham Road, Schaumburg, IL 60173-4965 (708) 330-9830.

The American Academy of Facial Plastic and Reconstructive Surgery 1110 Vermont Avenue, NW, Suite 220, Washington, DC 20005-3522 (202) 842-4500.

American Academy of Orthopedic Surgeons 6300 N. River Road, Rosemont, IL 60018-4262 (847) 823-7186.

American Association of Naturopathic Physicians P.O. Box 20386, Seattle, WA 98102 (206) 323-7610.

American Association of Sex Educators, Counselors and Therapists (AASECT) P.O. Box 238, Mount Vernon, IA 52314-0238 (319) 895-8407.

American Cancer Society, Inc. (ACS), National Headquarters 1599 Clifton Road, NE, Altanta, GA 30329 (800) ACS-2345, (800) 227-2345.

American College of Obstetricians and Gynecologists (ACOG) 409 12th Street, Washington, DC 20024 (202) 638-5577.

American Diabetic Association (ADA) 216 West Jackson Blvd., Suite 800, Chicago, IL 60606 (312) 899-0040.

American Heart Association 7272 Greenville Avenue, Dallas, TX 75231 (214) 373-6300.

American Holistic Medical Association 4101 Lake Boone Trail, Suite 201, Raleigh, NC 27607 (919) 787-5181.

American Holistic Nurses Association 4101 Lake Boone Trail, Suite 201, Raleigh, NC 27607 (919) 787-5181

American Society of Geriatric Physicians, 5600 South Quebec, Suite 109A, Englewood, CO 80111 (303) 779-4833.

Arthritis Foundation 1314 Spring Street, NW, Atlanta, GA 30309 (800) 283-7800.

Cancer Information Service, Office of Cancer Communications, Building 31, Room 10A24, Bethesda, MD 20892 (800) 4-CAN-CER, (800) 422-6237.

Cancer Research Institute 12011 San Vicente Blvd., Los Angeles, CA 90049 (310) 471-2720.

Citizens for Health P.O. Box 2260, Boulder, CO 80306 (800) 357-2211.

Health Resource Center 109 Holly Crescent, Suite 201, Virginia Beach, VA 23541 (804) 422-9022.

Institute for Noetic Sciences 475 Gate Five Road, Suite 300, Sausalito, CA 94965 (415) 331-5650.

International Association of Healthcare Practitioners - 1995 Directory. IAHP, 11211 Prosperity Farms Rd., D-325, Palm Beach Gardens, FL 33410.

International Foundation for Homeopathy P.O.Box 7, Edmonds, WA 98020 (206) 776-4147.

International Society for the Study of Subtle Energies and Energy Medicine 356 Goldco Circle, Golden, CO 80403-1347 (303) 278-2228.

National Arthritis and Musculoskeletal and Skin Disease Information Box AMS, 9000 Rockville Pike, Bethesda, MD 20892 (301) 495-4484.

National Heart, Lung and Blood Institute 9000 Rockville Pike, Bethesda, MD 20892 (301) 496-4236.

National Center for Homeopathy 801 North Fairfax Street, Suite 306, Alexandria, VA 22314 (703) 548-7790.

National Depressive and Manic-Depressive Association 730 N. Franklin St., Suite 501, Chicago, IL 60610 (800) 826-3632.

National Institute of Neurological Disorders and Stroke (NINDS) P.O. Box 5801, Bethesda, MD 20824 (800) 352-9424.

National Kidney and Urologic Diseases Information Clearinghouse (NKUDIC), 3 Info Way, Bethesda, MD 20892-3580 (301) 654-4415.

National Menopause Foundation, Inc. 222 SW 36th Terrace, Gainesville, FL 32607 (904) 372-7941.

National Osteoporosis Foundation 1150 17th St., NW, Suite 500, Washington, DC 20036 (800) 223-9994.

National Wellness Coalition; Contact: Janet Smith P.O. Box 3778, Washington, DC 20007-0278 (202) 333-1638.

National Women's Health Network 1325 G Street, NW, Washington, DC 20005 (202) 347-1140.

North American Menopause Society c/o P.O. Box 9452, Cleveland, OH 44101 (216) 844-8748 1(800) 774-5342, website www.meno-pause.org.

Office on Women's Health 200 Independence Ave., SW, Washington, DC 20201 (202) 690-7650.

Shealy Institute (pain, stress, depression management clinic) 1328 East Evergreen St., Springfield, MO 65648 (417) 865-5940.

The Skin Cancer Foundation 245 Fifth Avenue, Suite 2402, New York, NY 10016 (212) 725-5176.

ALTERNATIVE PHARMACIES

These pharmacies offer micronized progesterone, estriol, and estradiol as an estrogen replacement choice, micronized testosterone, DHEA and many other alternative products. Some of the companies are able to customize various strengths and combinations.

Bajamar Women's Health Center , 9609 Deilman Rock Island, St Louis, MO 63132 (800) 255-8025

Belmar Pharmacy, 12860 West Cedar Dr., #210, Lakewood, CO 80228 (800) 525-9473

Bezwecken Women's Health Products, 12525 South West 3rd Street Beaverton, OR 97005 (800) 743-2256

College Pharmacy, 833 North Tejon, Colorado Springs, CO 80903 (800) 888-9358

REFERENCES

Books:

Aburdene, P., and J. Naisbitt. 1992. *Megatrends for Women.* New York: Villard Books–Random House, Inc.

Alexander, Jo [et al.]. 1991. *Women and Aging: An Anthology* by Women. Corvallis, OR: Calyx Books.

Almaas, A. H. 1986. Essence: *The Diamond Approach to Inner Realization.* York Beach, Maine: Samuel Weiser, Inc.

————. 1990. *The Pearl Beyond Price.* Berkeley: Diamond Books.

American Medical Association. 1989. *Encyclopedia of Medicine.* New York: Random House, Inc.

Barbach, Lonnie, Ph.D. 1994. *The Erotic Edge: Erotica for Couples.* New York: Dutton.

————. 1994. *The Pause: Positive Approaches to Menopause.* New York: The Penguin Group.

————. 1984. For Each Other: *Sharing Sexual Intimacy.* New York: Signet.

Barbach, Lonnie, Ph.D., with David Geisinger. 1993. Going the Distance: Finding and Keeping Lifelong Love. New York: Plume.

Barnes, Broda O., M.D. and Lawrence Galton. 1976. *Hypothyroidism: The Unsuspected Illness.* New York: Harper Collins.

Berne, Katrina, 1995. *Running on Empty — The Complete Guide to Chronic Fatigue Syndrome.* Alameda, CA: Hunter House.

Boston Women's Health Book Collective. 1992. *The New Our Bodies, Ourselves.* New York: Simon & Schuster, Inc.

Brody, Jane. 1992. *Jane Brody's Good Food Gourmet.* New York: Bantam Books.

————. 1988. *Jane Brody's Nutrition Book.* Rev. ed. New York: W.W. Norton & Co.–Bantam Books.

————. 1983. *Jane Brody's The New York Times Guide to Personal Health.* New York: New York Times.

Carper, Jean. 1988. *The Food Pharmacy: Dramatic New Evidence That Food Is Your Best Medicine.* New York: Bantam Books.

Cherniske, Stephen, M.S. 1996. *The DHEA Breakthrough.* New York: Random House.

Chopra, Deepak, M.D. 1993. *Ageless Body, Timeless Mind.* New York: Harmony Books.

———. 1991. *Perfect Health.* New York: Harmony Books.

Daley, Rosie. 1991. *In the Kitchen with Rosie.* New York: Alfred A. Knopf.

Dossey, Larry, M.D. 1993. *Healing Words: The Power of Prayer & the Practice of Medicine.* San Francisco: Harper San Francisco.

———. 1989. *Recovering the Soul: A Scientific and Spiritual Search.* New York: Bantam Books.

Eliot, Robert S., and Dennis L. Breo. 1989. *Is It Worth Dying For? How to Make Stress Work for You, Not Against You.* Rev. ed. New York: Bantam Books.

Farrell-Kingsley, Kathy, and the editors of Woman's Day Magazine. 1995. *Woman's Day Cookbook.* New York: Penguin.

Gaby, Alan R., M.D. 1994. *Preventing and Reversing Osteoporosis: What You Can Do About Bone Loss.* Rocklin, CA: Prima Publishing.

Graedon, Joe, and Teresa Graedon, Ph.D. 1995. *The People's Guide to Deadly Drug Interactions.* New York: St. Martin's Press.

Greenwood, Sadja, M.D. 1992. *Menopause, Naturally.* Volcano, CA: Volcano Press.

Healy, Bernadine, M.D. 1995. *A New Prescription for Women's Health.* New York: Penguin.

Helgesen, Sally. 1995. *The Female Advantage.* New York: Doubleday.

———. 1995. *The Webb of Inclusion.* New York: Doubleday.

Inlander, Charles B., and the staff of the People's Medical Society. 1993. *Good Operations — Bad Operations.* New York: Viking.

Kenley, Joan, Ph.D. 1989. *Voice Power — A Breakthrough Method to Enhance Your Speaking Voice.* New York: Henry Holt and Co.

Kornfield, Jack. 1993. *A Path With Heart: A Guide Through the Perils and Promises of Spiritual Life*. New York: Bantam Books.

Kramer, Peter D. 1993. *Listening to Prozac*. New York: Viking Penguin.

Lamm, Steven, M.D. and Gerald Secor Couzens. 1995. *Thinner at Last*. New York: Simon & Schuster.

Lobo, Rogerio A. 1994. *Treatment of the Postmenopausal Woman: Basic and Clinical Aspects*. (For health advisors) New York: Raven Press.

Moffitt, Perry-Lynn. 1992. *A Silent Sorrow: Pregnancy Loss*. New York: Dell Books.

Moore, Thomas. 1992. *Care of the Soul*. New York: Harper Collins Publishers, Inc.

Nachtigall, Lila E., M.D., and Joan Rattner Heilman. 1991. *Estrogen*. New York: Harper Perennial.

Northrup, Christiane, M.D. 1994. *Women's Bodies, Women's Wisdom: Creating Physical and Emotional Health and Healing*. New York: Bantam Books.

Notelovitz, Morris, M.D., and Diana Tonnessen. 1993. *Menopause & Midlife Health*. First Edition. New York: St. Martin's Press.

Ornish, Dean, M.D. 1990. *Dr. Dean Ornish's Program for Reversing Heart Disease*. New York: Ballantine Books-Random House, Inc.

Perry, Susan, and Katherine Walker, M.D. 1992. *Natural Menopause*. Reading, Massachusetts: Addison-Wesley Publishing Co.

Rapoport, Alan, M.D. and Fred Sheftell, M.D. 1995. *Headache Relief for Women*. New York: Little Brown.

Remen, Rachel Naomi, M.D. 1994. *Kitchen Table Wisdom*. New York: Riverhead Books.

Ricketson, Susan Cooley, Ph.D. 1989. *The Dilemma of Love*. Deerfield Beach, Florida: Health Communications, Inc.

Rosoff, Ilene and The Launch Pad Contributors. 1995. *The Woman Source Catalog & Review: "Tools for Connecting the Community of Women."* Berkeley, CA: Celestial Arts.

Seagal, Sandra, and David Horne. 1996. Human Dynamics and the Life of Organizations. Boston: Pegasus Communications.

Sears, Barry, Ph.D. 1997. *Mastering the Zone.* New York: Regan Books.

———. 1995. *The Zone.* New York: HarperCollins.

Sheehy, Gail. 1995. *New Passages.* New York: Random House.

———. 1992. *The Silent Passage: Menopause.* New York: Random House.

Siegel, Bernie, M.D. 1986. *Love, Medicine & Miracles.* New York: Harper and Row.

———. 1986. *Peace, Love & Healing.* New York: Harper and Row.

Ullman, Dana, M.D. 1991. *Discovering Homeopathy.* Revised Edition. Berkeley: North Atlantic Books.

Utian, Wulf H., M.D., Ph.D., and Ruth S. Jacobowitz. 1992. *Managing Your Menopause.* New York: Simon & Schuster.

Weed, Susan S. 1992. *Menopausal Years: The Wise Woman Way.* New York: Ash Tree Publishing.

Witkin, Georgia, Ph.D. 1984, 1991. *The Female Stress Syndrome.* New York: Newmarket Press.

Zukav, Gary. 1990. *The Seat of the Soul.* New York: Fireside.

Magazines:

Health, Time Publishing Ventures, Inc., 301 Howard St., Ste. 1800, San Francisco, CA 94105.

Intuition Magazine, P.O. Box 460773, San Francisco, CA 94146.

Natural Health, Boston Common Press Limited Partnership, 17 Station Street, Box 1200, Brookline Village, MA 02147.

Nature, Nature Publishing Company, 65 Bleeker Street, New York, NY 10012.

Prevention, Rodale Press, Inc., 33 E. Minor Street, Emmaus, PA 18098.

Women's Health & Menopause Newsletters:

A Friend Indeed, A Friend Indeed Publications, Inc., Box 515, Place du Parc Station, Montreal, Quebec H2W 2P1.

Harvard Women's Health Watch, P.O. Box 420234, Palm Coast, FL 32142.

Menopause News, 2074 Union St., San Francisco, CA 94123.

Midlife Woman, Midlife Women's Network, 5129 Logan Avenue South, Minneapolis, MN 55419-1019.

Women's Health Access, P.O. Box 9690, Madison, WI 53715.

Women's Health Connections, P.O. Box 6338, Madison, WI 53716-0338.

Journals & Health Publications:

AARP Bulletin, American Association of Retired Persons, 601 E Street NW, Washington, D.C. 20049.

The Johns Hopkins Medical Letter: Health After fifty, 550 North Broadway, Suite 110, Johns Hopkins, Baltimore, MD 21205-2011.

Menopause Management: An Educational Publication Endorsed by the North American Menopause Society, The Conwood Group, Inc., 9 Mt. Pleasant Turnpike, Denville, NJ 07834.

Menopause: The Journal of the North American Menopause Society, Raven Press, 1185 Avenue of the Americas, New York, NY 10036.

Mind & Energy Newsletter, Linda Prout, M.S., c/o Claremont Resort & Spa, 41 Tunnel Road, Berkeley, CA 94623.

Women's Health Digest, Women to Woman America, 222 SW 36 Terrace, Gainesville, FL 32607.

INDEX

Listings do not include the *Diagnostic Questionnaire,*
Check-Up Schedule, or *References, Resources, & Glossary.*

ABOUT THE AUTHOR

Whose Body Is It Anyway is a book Dr. Joan Kenley, wellness coach, author, and psychologist, had to write. At mid-life, having faced her own life-threatening and difficult-to-diagnose health problems, she became a crusader for women's health.

Dr. Kenley, who has served on the leadership board for JKF University and is the Director of Personal Growth Programs for Core Leadership Development, speaks before national audiences, co-facilitates a healthcare CEO forum, and designs one-of-a-kind wellness programs. She has been a consultant, trainer, and personal coach for twenty years.

Dr. Kenley educates women to take charge of their choices and to think differently about their bodies. Her work focuses on full-spectrum health drawing on her rich research and experience in physical, emotional, mental, and spiritual perspectives. She has appeared on *Dateline, 20/20,* CNN, *Good Morning America,* and *The Oprah Winfrey Show* among others, and has been featured on countless radio shows and in many national publications including *The New York Times Magazine, Reader's Digest, Health,* and *Allure.*

Prior to her work as a psychologist and health professional, Dr. Kenley explored the healing aspects of the speaking voice. Her acclaimed book, *Voice Power,* details her innovative six-step BodyVoice Method™ which improves the sound of the voice while empowering one's personal and professional life. Her work in broadcasting has led her to become known worldwide for her warm, friendly "voice" on such recognizable voicemail and digitized phone products as Pacific Bell Message Center, NYNEX Information Services, Northern Telecom Meridian Mail, and American Personal Communications Sprint Spectrum.

Dr. John C. Arpels. M.D, is a practitioner of gynecology and menopausal medicine. He is a founding member of the North American Menopause Society; Associate Clinical Professor, U.C. San Francisco, Department of Obstetrics, Gynecology & Reproductive Services.

DATE DUE

Demco